ALLE ZEIT WACH
1842

Iwao Honjo

Eustachian Tube and Middle Ear Diseases

With 182 Figures, Some of Them in Color

Springer-Verlag
Tokyo Berlin Heidelberg New York London Paris

Iwao Honjo
Professor and Chairman
Department of Otolaryngology
Faculty of Medicine
Kyoto University
54 Shogoin Kawaharacho
Sakyo-ku, Kyoto, 606 Japan

ISBN-13: 978-4-431-68289-9 e-ISBN-13: 978-4-431-68287-5
DOI: 10.1007/978-4-431-68287-5

Library of Congress Cataloging-in-Publication Data

Honjō, Iwao, 1935– . Eustachian tube and middle ear diseases/Iwao Honjō.
p. cm. Includes bibliographies and index. ISBN-13: 978-4-431-68289-9
Germany: est) 1. Middle ear—Diseases. 2. Eustachian tube—Diseases.
I. Title. [DNLM: 1. Ear, Middle—physiopathology. 2. Eustachian Tube—
physiopathology. 3. Otitis Media with Effusion. WV 230 H773e] RF220.H66
1988 617.8′4—dc19 DNLM/DLC for Library of Congress

Softcover reprint of the hardcover 1st edition 1988

Typesetting: Asco Trade Typesetting Ltd, Hong Kong

Preface

The relationship between the eustachian tube and middle ear diseases is both an old and a new clinical problem, which should not be overlooked by the otolaryngologist. Earlier investigators such as Politzer, Bezold, Zaufal, and Zöllner revealed a close relationship between these two organs. More recently, the aerodynamic studies of Ingelstedt et al. and the investigations on the eustachian tube and the middle ear by Bluestone and his colleagues were innovative in the research into this area. In Japan also, a number of achievements in this field have been made by Takahara, Kawamoto, and Kumazawa.

I started my career studying cleft palate, then turned my interest to the eustachian tube, and became involved in middle ear problems. Through these investigations, I came across a number of questions such as why the incidence of otitis media is high in individuals with cleft palate and whether the hydropus ex vacuo theory is still applicable to the pathogenesis of otitis media with effusion.

I entitle this volume "The Eustachian Tube and Middle Ear Diseases" because the eustachian tube is considered to participate in middle ear diseases more actively than is generally estimated. A large number of patients with ear diseases, including those with cleft palate or nasopharyngeal carcinoma, were examined by as many approaches as possible to clarify the etiology, pathology, and even prognosis of middle ear diseases in relation to the eustachian tube.

Many of the studies in this volume, however, are not conclusive but still open for discussion. I feel like I am viewing a distant mountain range from the foothills. I sincerely hope that this volume will be a step toward further advancement in our knowledge about the eustachian tube and middle ear diseases.

I would like to express my sincere gratitude to my colleagues at the department: Dr. M. Hayashi, Dr. H. Takahashi, Dr. Y. Tasaka, Dr. Y. Naito, Dr. H. Sato, Dr. A. Fujita, and Dr. K. Mori, for their collaboration in preparing this book. I also extend my thanks to Professor T. Hsieh, Department of Otolaryngology, National Taiwan University, Professor K. Hoshino, Department of Anatomy, Kyoto

University, Emeritus Professor K. Torizuka, Department of Nuclear Medicine, Kyoto University and Prof. O. Tanaka, Department of Anatomy, Shimane Medical University for their warm assistance. I also thank Dr. Y. Naito's cooperation in preparing the manuscript and Ms. S. Date for typing.

July 1988 IWAO HONJO

Table of Contents

Chapter 1
Development of Auditory Organs from Embryological Viewpoint

In diseases of the middle ear such as otitis media with effusion (OME), the auditory organs are, so to speak, immersed in fluid. Magnetic resonance imaging (MRI) clearly depicts this condition in a patient with OME, whose mastoid air cells and even the eustachian tube are filled with fluid, resembling that of a fetus immersed in the amniotic fluid in the uterus (Fig. 1.1).

The process of embryonic development reproduces, in a sense, the long history of human evolution in the 38 weeks of fetal life. This ontogenic process of the embryo indicates something of human phylogenesis. To investigate the development of the auditory organs, especially the eustachian tube, from this perspective, human embryos were examined under the light microscope. Serial sections, 8 μm thick, of 12 human embryos at a fetal age of 6–7 weeks were stained with hematoxylin-eosin and azan.

The inner ear develops from ectodermal thickenings (auditory placodes) in the lateral portion of the rhombencephalon at some distance from the middle ear

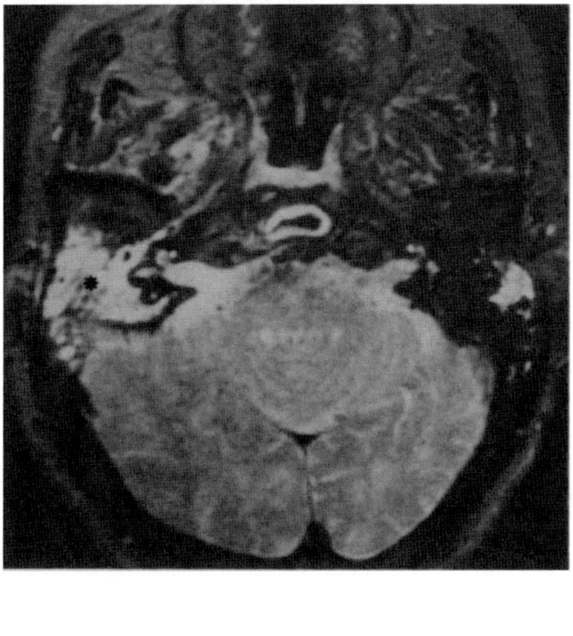

Fig. 1.1. Magnetic resonance imaging of otitis media with effusion. Mastoid air cells (*) and eustachian tube are completely filled with effusion

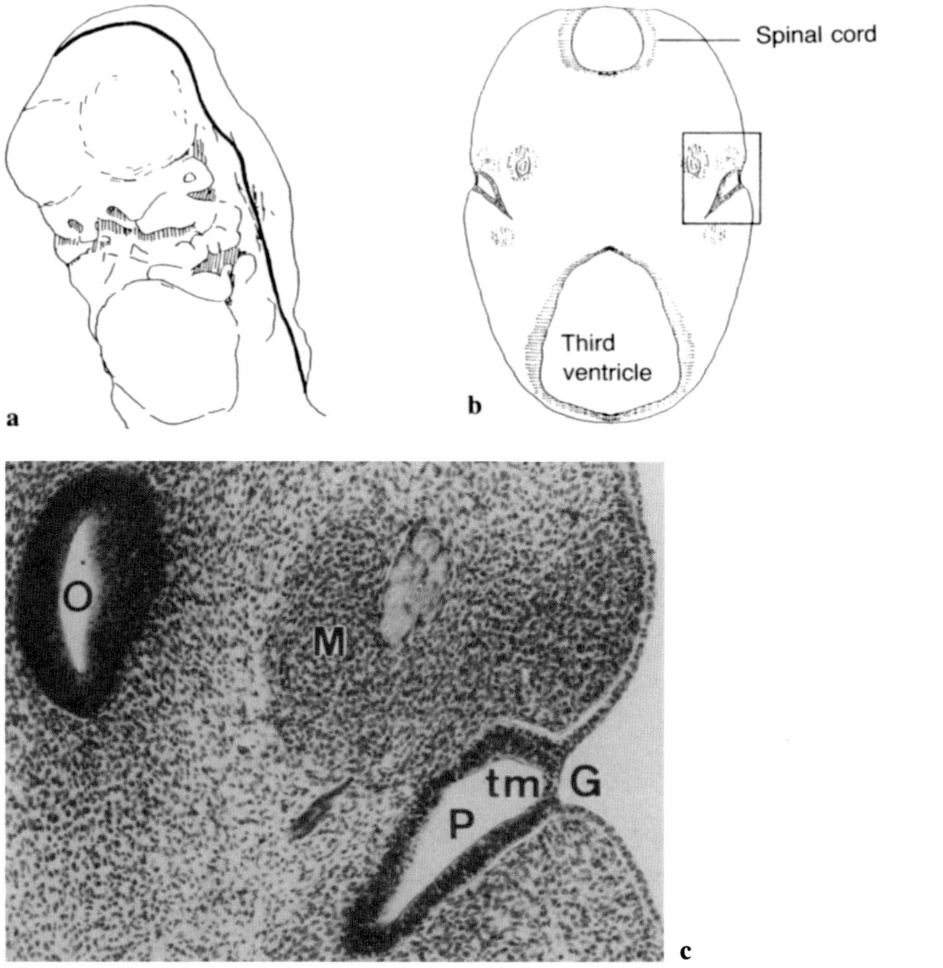

Fig. 1.2a–c. **a** Cutting plane. **b** Cross section. **c** Cross section of a human embryo at 6th week. *P* first pharyngeal pouch, *G* first branchial groove, *tm* primordial tympanic membrane, *M* aggregations of mesenchymal cells comprising primordia of auditory ossicles, *O* otic vesicle

primordium and forms otic vesicles, which are the prototype of the inner ear (Fig. 1.2). Concerning the middle ear, the tympanic cavity and eustachian tube start as the first pharyngeal pouch, which rapidly extends laterally and comes into contact with the first branchial groove, the rudiment of the external auditory meatus, in the 6th embryonal week. The pharyngeal pouch and branchial groove then become separated by the thin membranous structure of the primordial tympanic membrane. At this time, the primordia of the auditory ossicles are observed adjacent to the first branchial groove as aggregations of mesenchymal cells, but they are still separated from the rudiment of the inner ear (otic vescicle).

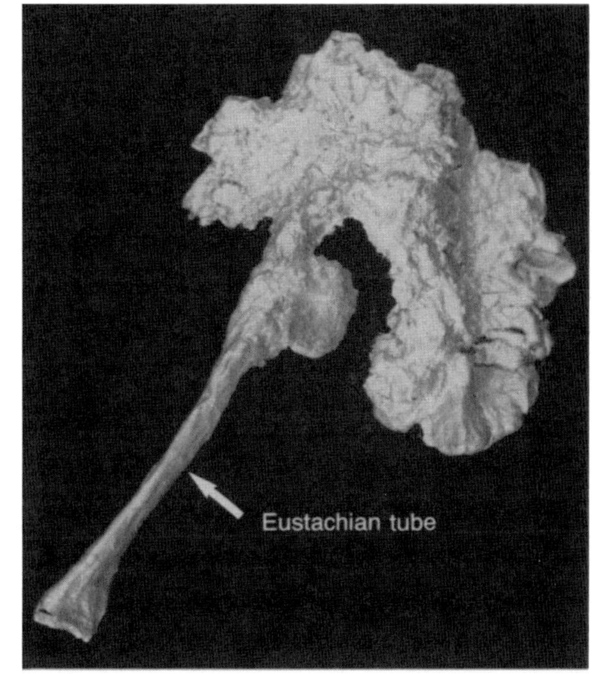

Fig. 1.3. Mold of left eustachian tube and mastoid air cells. Eustachian tube ventilates a large air-filled cavity located at its end

A thin tube of the first branchial groove remains in the same form to become the eustachian tube, and its lateral portion enlarges to develop into the tympanic cavity. Then, two different parts of the ear, namely the inner ear of ectodermal origin (otic vesicle) and the middle ear of mesenchymal and ectodermal origin, fuse to form the auditory organs. This process is considered to reflect the adaptation that our aquatic ancestors made when they began living on land, retaining water in the inner ear. To conduct sound vibration efficiently to the inner ear, sensory cells surrounded by fluid, the air-filled cavity of the middle ear develops as a mechanical amplifier between the inner ear and the external world. Thus, the tympanic cavity developed from the first pharyngeal groove, with a connecting tube (eustachian tube) to the external air space. Consequently, the eustachian tube came to play an important role in maintaining the middle ear as an air-filled cavity (Fig. 1.3).

The middle ear is, thus, a newly developed structure in the evolution from aquatic to land animals and is filled with air like the lung. Although the auditory system of aquatic animals like sharks conducts the sound directly to the inner ear via water, an air-filled space has to mediate sound conduction in the human ear (Fig. 1.4). If the eustachian tube connecting the ear to the exterior is blocked or the middle ear becomes filled with fluid, the ear immediately loses its function as an auditory organ.

Thus, as a result of the evolutionary development from ancestors who carried water in the ear, the air-filled cavity of the middle ear cannot function without a canal (eustachian tube) for ventilation. Such an auditory organ in man is regarded in one sense as defective, though it is the result of an elaborate evolution-

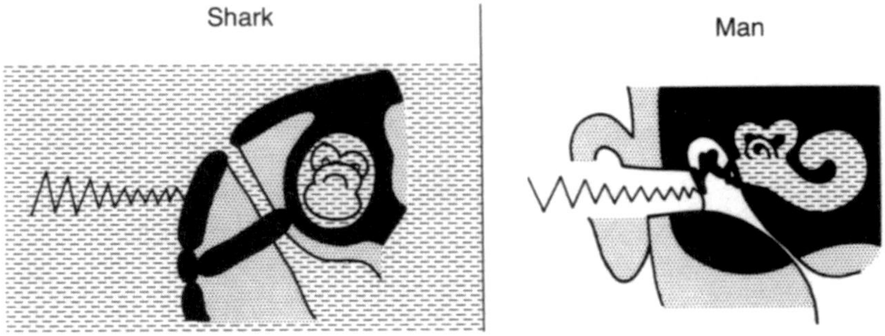

Fig. 1.4. Difference in auditory organs between aquatic and terrestrial creatures. *Shaded area* water

ary process for sound conduction. Failure to maintain the middle ear space in an air-filled condition, which is a kind of retrogression of the mammalian ear to an embryonic or aquatic stage, occurs in OME. This concept will be discussed in Chap. 5.

Summary of Chapter

Human embryos at a fetal age of 6–7 weeks were examined with respect to the differentiation of the auditory organ, and the relation between the inner and middle ear, including the eustachian tube, was investigated.

The air-filled cavity of the middle ear originated from the first branchial pouch to facilitate the conduction of sound vibrations in the air to the sensory cells of the inner ear, which are surrounded by fluid. The eustachian tube, which opens to the exterior, has an important function in maintaining the middle ear in an air-filled condition for better hearing.

Chapter 2
Three-Dimensional Reconstruction of Eustachian Tube and Related Muscles

Although the eustachian tube is a thin canal of only about 3.5 cm in length, connecting the ear with the nasopharynx, morphological examination of this organ is not easy because of its location deep in the cranium. A number of attempts have been made to visualize the eustachian tube by means of, for example, histological sections of the tube (Graves and Edwards 1944), molding of the tubal lumen (Aschan 1955), contrast roentgenograms (Welin 1947), and endoscopy of the tube (Ohsawa and Nanjo 1952).

When the eustachian tube is viewed along its long axis, the difficulty of visualizing it as a whole becomes apparent because it extends from the pharyngeal orifice, closely surrounded posterolaterally by muscles and connective tissue, toward the bony part of the temporal bone (Fig. 2.1). In addition to the eustachian tube itself, the tubal cartilage and tensor and levator veli palatini muscles are closely related to the function of the tube.

In order to obtain clear images of the tube with the surrounding structures, a three-dimensional image was reconstructed by computer graphics from two-dimensional data of serial sections of the tube. A few studies of three-dimensional reconstruction of the eustachian tube have been made (Siegel et al. 1983, 1985).

2.1 Preparation of Serial Sections of Eustachian Tube

To obtain data for computer graphics, serial sections of the eustachian tube were first prepared. The temporal bone, including the eustachian tube, of an adult woman with no history of ear disease was embedded in polyester resin and cut into serial sections vertical to the axis of the tube. Sections, 400–500 μm thick, were prepared by a hard-tissue cutting machine (MC-4110, Maruto, Tokyo, Japan) and then ground to a thickness of 200 μm without decalcification. The sections were stained with toluidine blue and hematoxylin and eosin to differentiate clearly tissues such as the cartilage, muscle, bone, and glandular tissue (Fig. 2.2).

By this procedure, the specimens could be obtained after about 1 month, and the staining was no less satisfactory than with specimens prepared by celloidin embedding, which requires at least 6 months. A total of 28 serial sections pre-

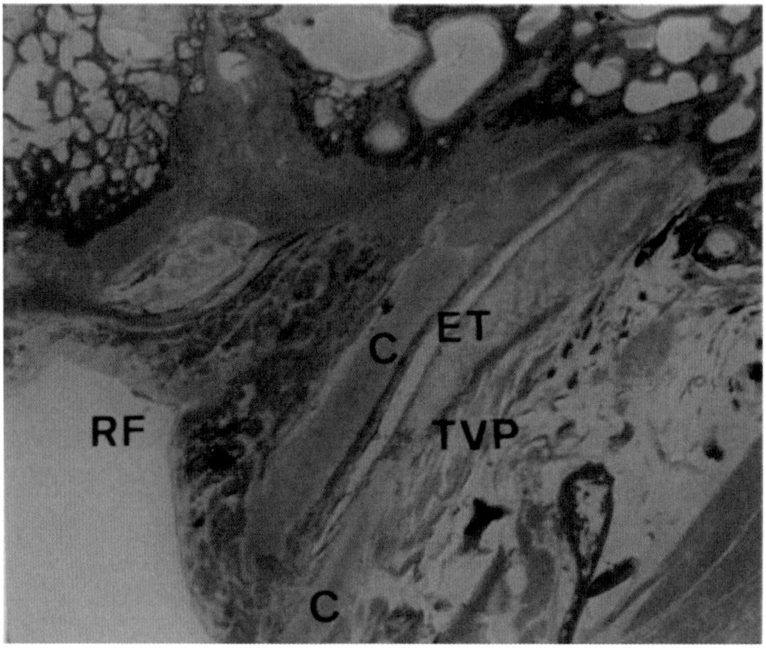

Fig. 2.1. Horizontal section of the left eustachian tube. *ET* eustachian tube, *C* tubal cartilage, *TVP* tensor veli palatini muscle, *RF* lateral pharyngeal recess (Rosenmüller's fossa)

pared at intervals of 1.2 mm, which were adequate for structural evaluation of the tube, were used to obtain the basic data for the three-dimensional representation of the eustachian tube with its surrounding tissues.

2.2 Three-Dimensional Computer Graphics of Eustachian Tube

The serial sections were traced by a graphic digitizer (MPC-8501, NEC, Tokyo, Japan), and two-dimensional xy-data were input into a personal computer (PC9801VM2, NEC, Tokyo, Japan). Figure 2.3 shows the input data arranged in order. Four sections containing the mucosa of the tubal lumen, tubal cartilage, the tensor palatini muscle, and the levator palatini muscle were approximated with 25-angle polygons. Three-dimensional data were then obtained by calculating the z-axis values from the slice interval; coordinate conversion and two-dimensional projection were carried out from these data and the coordinate data of an arbitrary view. A wire-frame model was then drawn by connecting corresponding points, considering the continuity of the sections. In this process, hidden structures were shaded by the z-buffer method (perspective visualization).

The results are as shown in Figs. 2.4 and 2.5, the former being an upper anterolateral view and the latter an upper posterolateral view of the left eustachian tube. The figures clearly illustrate the spacial relations between the osseous and

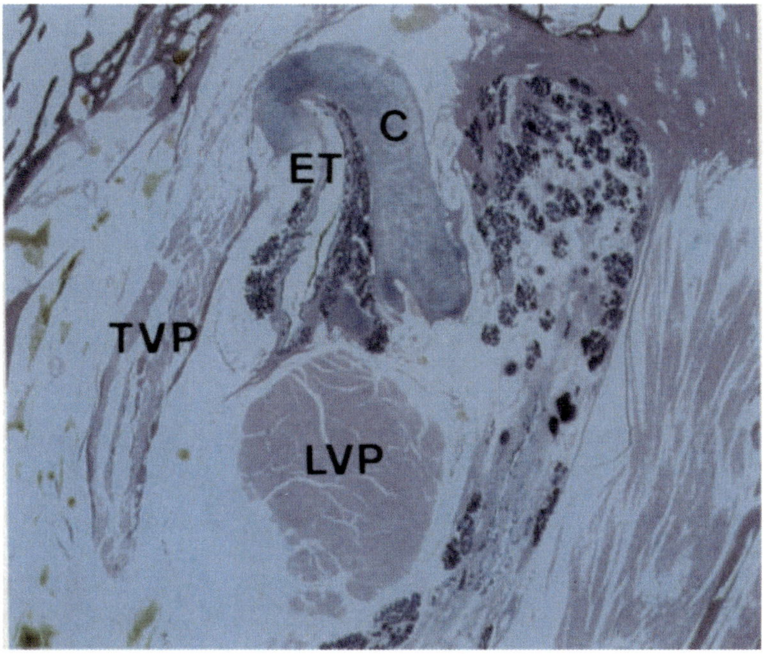

Fig. 2.2. Vertical section of the right eustachian tube in its mid-portion. *ET* eustachian tube, *C* tubal cartilage, *TVP* tensor veli palatini muscle, *LVP* levator veli palatini muscle

cartilaginous portions of the eustachian tube, and also those among the tubal cartilage, tensor palatini muscle, and levator palatini muscle.

Using computer graphics, the tubal cartilage can be removed, as in Fig. 2.6, and both the tensor palatini and levator palatini muscles can be erased from Fig. 2.5, as shown in Fig. 2.7. The lateral plate of the tubal cartilage is slightly protruded in the central third, indicating the site of insertion of the tensor palatini muscle. Although the levator palatini muscle has been considered to run parallel with the eustachian tube, the graphic images show that only the distal half of the muscle is in contact with the eustachian tube and the proximal half is not in contact, being separated by the C-shaped tubal cartilage surrounding the tubal lumen. These images also indicate that the levator muscle has little effect on opening of the tube.

As shown in Figs. 2.7 and 2.8, the tubal lumen is narrowed at the proximal end of the tubal cartilage, constituting the isthmus of the eustachian tube.

The tensor palatini muscle, the most important muscle for opening the eustachian tube, covers the anterior three-fourths of the tubal cartilage (Fig. 2.5), though its anterior portion arises from the skull base. These portions lacking contact with the tubal cartilage can be removed, as in Fig. 2.9. This graphic image suggests that the tensor palatini muscle is effective only in the posterior one-fourth of the tube, which indicates that the function of this muscle in tubal opening is greatest in this area.

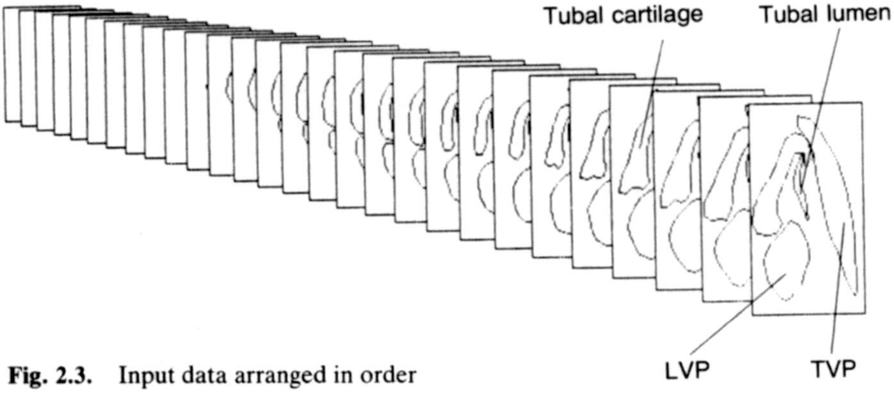

Fig. 2.3. Input data arranged in order

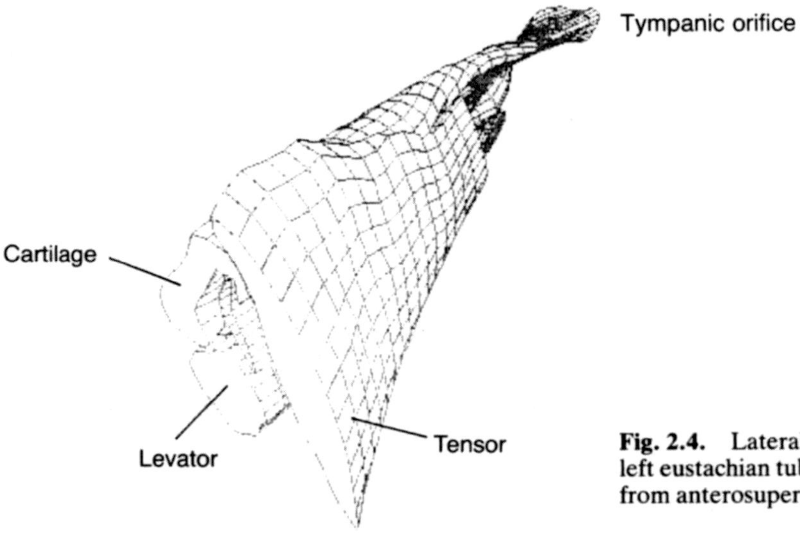

Fig. 2.4. Lateral view of a left eustachian tube system from anterosuperior direction

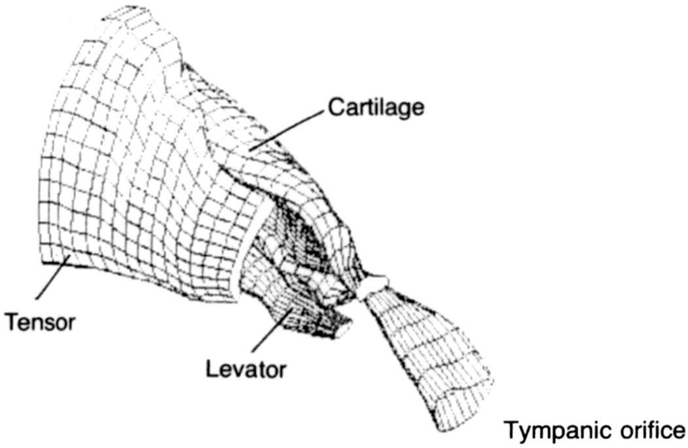

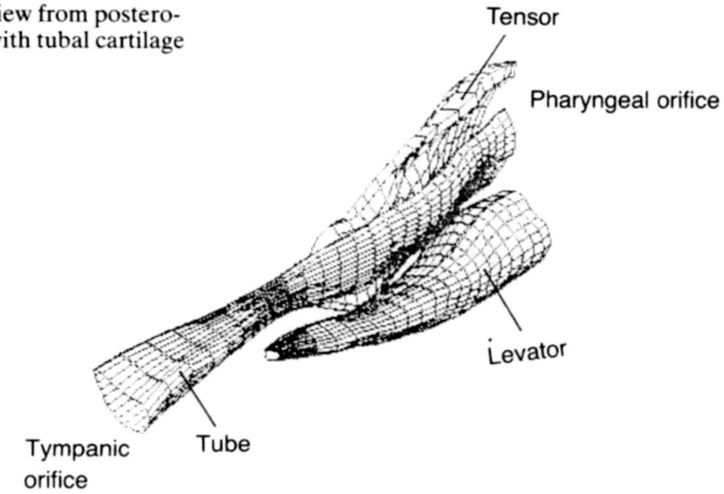

Fig. 2.6. Medial view from postero-superior direction with tubal cartilage removed

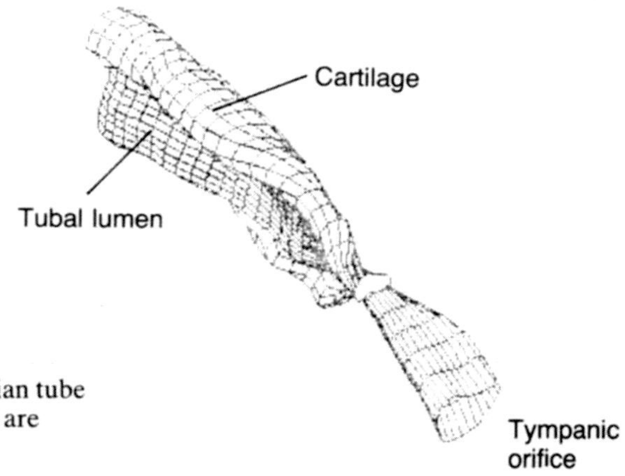

Fig. 2.7. Lateral view of eustachian tube and tubal cartilage. Tubal muscles are removed

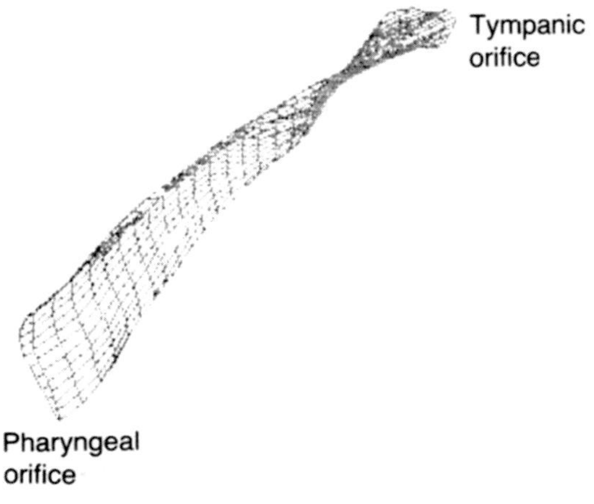

Fig. 2.8. Lateral view of tubal lumen alone

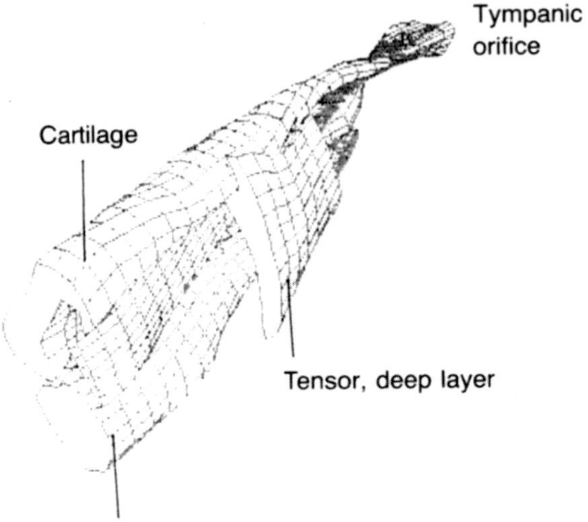

Fig. 2.9. Eustachian tube after removal of superficial layer of tensor veli palatini muscle originating from cranial bone

2.3 Summary of Chapter

Two-dimensional data obtained from serial sections of the eustachian tube were converted into three-dimensional images by a computer. This allowed morphological evaluation of the eustachian tube from various angles and facilitated better understanding of the relation between morphology and function of the eustachian tube.

References

Aschan G (1955) The anatomy of the eustachian tube with regard to its function. Acta Soc Med Upsal 60:131–149

Graves GO, Edwards LF (1944) The eustachian tube: A review of its descriptive, microscopic, topographic and clinical anatomy. Arch Otolaryngol 39:359–397

Ohsawa R, Nanjo S (1952) Visual examination of the pharyngeal orifice of the eustachian tube using nasopharyngoscope. Jibi Inkoka 24:465–483 (in Japanese with English abstract)

Siegel MI, Todhunter JS, Doyle WJ, Rood SR (1983) Computer reconstruction of eustachian tube anatomy. Ann Otol Rhinol Laryngol 92 (Suppl 107):10

Siegel MI, Todhunter JX, Sadler-Kimes D (1985) New methodology for unbiased computer reconstruction of histologic preparations. Ann Otol Rhinol Laryngol 94 (Suppl 120):11–12

Welin S (1947) On the radiological examination of the eustachian tube in cases of chronic otitis. Acta Radiol 28:95–103

Chapter 3
Function of Eustachian Tube

During swallowing and yawning, the eustachian tube ventilates the middle ear to equalize its pressure with that of the atmosphere. The clearance function of the tube becomes important when fluid accumulates in the middle ear, as in the case of otitis media with effusion. Thus, two different functions of the eustachian tube serve to maintain the normal condition of the ear.

Concerning the ventilation function of the eustachian tube, it opens only for a short time during swallowing or yawning. One becomes aware of this type of tubal function in an airplane as a sudden relief of the feeling of compression in the ear or hearing loss after swallowing. In this way, the eustachian tube regulates the middle ear by normalizing pressure to maintain good hearing.

The other function of the tube is clearance of fluid in the middle ear, which causes sensation of fullness in the ear and hearing impairment. Drainage of such fluid into the pharynx at an early stage is an essential function of the tube to maintain the ear in a normal working condition. The clearance function of the eustachian tube may be divided into muscular and ciliary functions. In contrast to the ciliary function, the muscular or pumplike activity of the eustachian tube in expelling a foreign substance from the ear remains obscure.

In the following study, the mechanism of muscular drainage of fluid was investigated. Quantitative differences between muscular and ciliary clearance and the effects of viscosity of the middle ear effusion on these clearance abilities were also examined.

3.1 Muscles Opening the Eustachian Tube

The eustachian tube opens by contraction of the so-called tubal muscles during swallowing or yawning. Between the tensor veli palatini and levator veli palatini muscles, contraction of the tensor muscle only (Rich 1920; Holborow 1962) or the combined action of the tensor and levator muscles (Toynbee 1853; Politzer 1909; McMyn 1940; Zöllner 1942; Aschan 1955) have been considered to be responsible for opening the tube. Since the tensor muscle originates in the tubal cartilage and the levator runs parallel to the eustachian tube, these muscles are thought to be involved in the movement of the eustachian tube. The following experiments reveal how each of the muscles participates in the tubal opening and what muscle is primarily responsible for this movement.

3.1.1 Electric Stimulation of Tensor and Levator Muscles

Using dogs and monkeys, the tensor and levator muscles were contracted separately to determine the muscle responsible for opening the eustachian tube. Cantekin et al. (1979) induced contraction of these muscles by electric stimulation of the nerves innervating the muscles at the skull base. In our study, electric stimulation was applied directly to the muscles under general anesthesia of pentobarbital sodium (Nembutal). Bipolar needle electrodes were inserted into each muscle via the oral cavity. Positive pressure was applied to the middle ear through a perforation of the eardrum to detect the tubal opening by the sudden drop in pressure.

The pressure of the middle ear dropped suddenly when the tensor muscle was stimulated with relatively low electric potentials, indicating that this muscle opens the tube. In contrast, stimulation of the levator muscle produced no tubal opening, even at high potentials of electric stimulation (Fig. 3.1).

To summarize, the eustachian tube opened consistently upon tensor stimulation at a low electric potential (mean, 0.6 V), while the tube did not open upon stimulation of the levator up to 20 V, which was the maximum level of stimulation (Table 3.1). These findings indicate that the eustachian tube opens by contraction of the tensor muscle alone and not by that of the levator muscle.

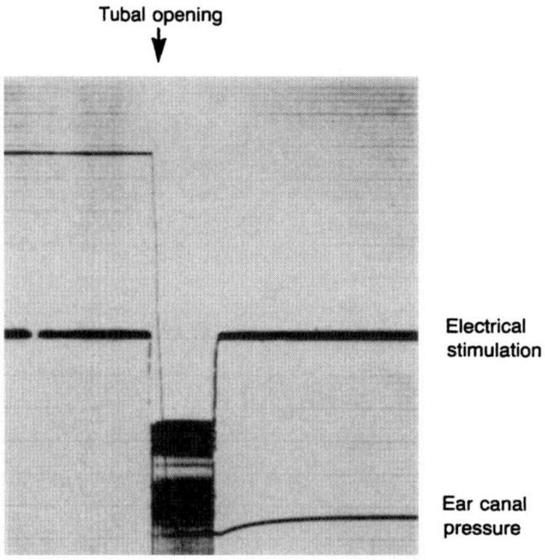

Fig. 3.1. Tubal opening caused by electric stimulation of tensor muscle

Table 3.1. Thresholds of the tensor (left column) and the levator (right column) stimulation for tubal opening

No.	Electrical stimulation	No.	Electrical stimulation
1	0.3 V	1	18.0 V <
2	0.4 V	2	18.0 V <
3	0.4 V	3	20.0 V <
4	0.5 V	4	20.0 V <
5	0.6 V	5	18.0 V <
6	1.0 V	6	20.0 V <
7	1.0 V		
mean	0.6 V		

3.1.2 Facilitatory Effect of Levator Muscle on Tubal Opening

The levator muscle has been thought to assist the tensor muscle in opening the eustachian tube. In accordance with this, contraction of the levator alone would not cause tubal opening, but the muscle would have a facilitatory effect on the opening by simultaneously contracting with the tensor muscle. This hypothesis was examined as follows.

First, the threshold of the tensor stimulation for tubal opening was determined (Fig. 3.2). In the dog shown in Fig. 3.2, the tube opened at 0.6 V and 0.7 V, but not at 0.5 V. Thus the threshold of tubal opening was considered to be 0.6 V. Then, simultaneously with the subthreshold tensor stimulation (0.5 V), high-voltage stimulation was applied to the levator muscle. If the levator helped the tensor in tubal opening, the tube would be expected to open. However, no tubal

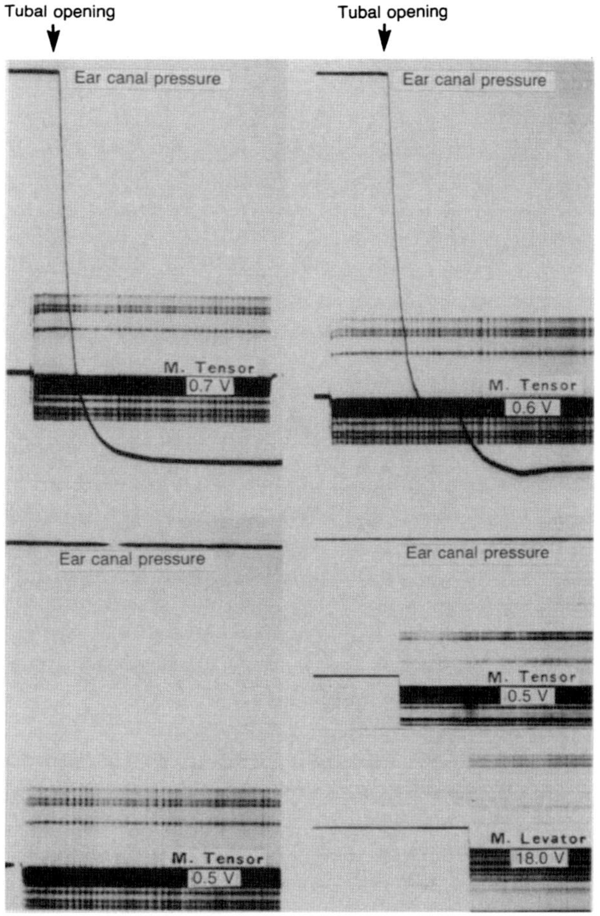

Fig. 3.2. Minimum threshold of tensor for tubal opening was determined to be 0.6 V (*upper row*). Simultaneous stimulation of tensor (using 0.5 V) and levator (using 18 V) produced no opening of tube (*lower right*)

opening occurred.

Thus, it was confirmed that the tensor muscle is the only muscle involved in opening the eustachian tube and that the levator muscle does not play even a facilitatory role in this function.

3.2 Opening Process of Eustachian Tube

Various attempts at observing the process of opening of the eustachian tube have been made, but they were often hampered by the deep location of the tube inside the head. Movement of the tube was observed roentgenographically in monkeys and humans.

3.2.1 Contrast X-Ray Study of Eustachian Tube

Using monkeys, the movement of the eustachian tube following electric stimulation of the tubal muscles was visualized roentgenographically. The animals were anesthetized by intravenous injection of Nembutal. Needle electrodes were inserted into the tensor and levator muscles through the mouth. Roentgenograms and cineroentgenograms of the eustachian tube were obtained by infusing the contrast medium into the middle ear through the perforated eardrum. By electric stimulation of each muscle, the effect of the muscle contraction on the tubal movement was observed.

First, it was confirmed that the eustachian tube opens due to contraction of the tensor muscle but closes upon cessation of the contraction. On the other hand, opening of the tube does not occur by contraction of the levator muscle (Fig. 3.3).

Detailed observation of the roentgenograms revealed that the contraction of the tensor produced a slight but definite tubal opening not only at the small area around the isthmus, but also along almost the entire cartilaginous part of the tube. By comparison of the tubal lumen before and during the tensor stimulation, it was noted that the tubal opening resulted from outward displacement of the lateral tubal wall, as shown in Fig. 3.4. The medial wall of the tube, by contrast, showed no movement. Stimulation of the levator muscle, however, did not cause any opening of the tube as a whole; it merely produced an inward movement of the tubal torus at the distal end of the tube. Consequently, the lumen of the pharyngeal orifice of the tube dilated into a funnel shape by the levator contraction (Fig. 3.5).

The roentgenographic findings that the levator produces no tubal opening coincide well with previous findings of manometric studies. The levator causes only a widening of the distal end of the tube, the pharyngeal orifice. In endoscopic observation of the tube orifice, care must be taken in this regard not to mistake the widening of the orifice for an opening of the tube.

Since two different muscles are related to the tube, its opening process has been regarded as being fairly complicated. However, the present study reveals that the tube opens in quite a simple way. The tensor muscle pulls the lateral wall of the tube, laterally and caudally, toward the hamulus to which the tensor is attached, while the levator dilates only the distal end around the pharyngeal orifice.

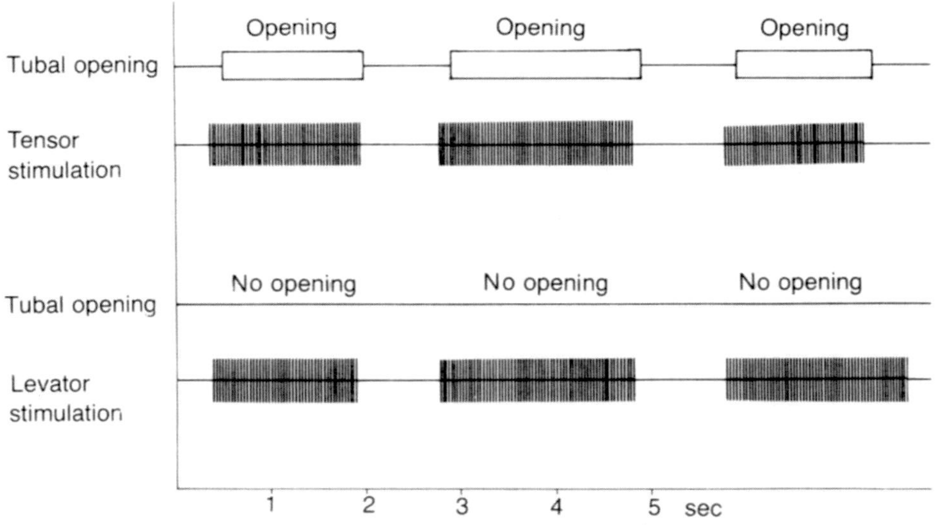

Fig. 3.3. Relation between muscle stimulation and tubal opening

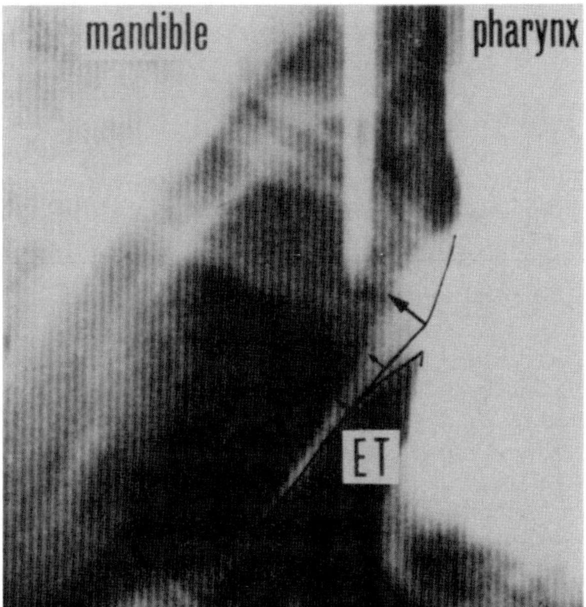

Fig. 3.4. Outward movement of tubal wall upon tensor stimulation. *Solid line* shows original position of tube, and *arrows* indicate outward displacement of the wall upon stimulation

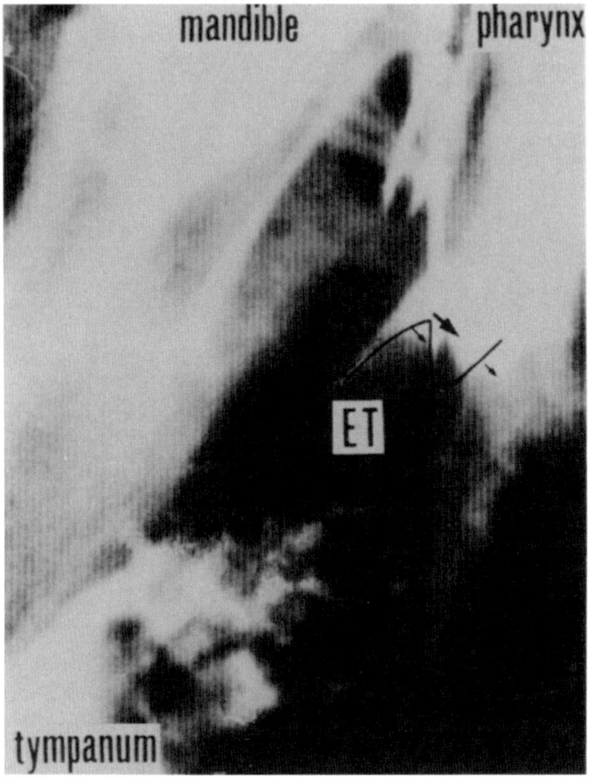

Fig. 3.5. Inward movement of right torus tubarius upon levator stimulation. *Solid* line shows original position of torus and *arrows* indicate its inward displacement

3.2.2 Roentgenographic Observation of Tubal Movement in Humans

The opening process of the tube during swallowing was examined roentgenographically in humans. In patients with a perforated eardrum, the tube was visualized by the instillation of contrast medium (iodamide) through the perforated eardrum. Cineroentgenograms of a vertical view of the tube during swallowing were taken at a speed of 24 frames/s.

Frame-by-frame analysis of the film revealed a difference of tubal movement at the distal (pharyngeal orifice) and proximal parts. First, the distal part of the tube near the pharyngeal orifice began to open in swallowing due to a marked inward movement of the torus tubarius. Just after dilatation of the pharyngeal orifice, the proximal part of the tube, comprising almost the entire cartilaginous section, opened for a short time. The degree of tubal opening was very slight and almost equal at all parts of the tube except the orifice.

The movement of the human eustachian tube described in this section is very similar to that seen with electric stimulation in monkeys; namely, there were two different processes of tubal opening at two parts of the tube: lateral pull of the tube by the tensor contraction and dilatation of the pharyngeal orifice by the levator contraction.

3.3 Muscular Clearance of Eustachian Tube

Fluid retained in the middle ear may be expelled partly by ciliary action in the tube, but quick and massive expulsion occurs by muscular or so-called pumping function of the tube. The following studies revealed which muscle mainly contributes to muscular clearance and how this function is performed. Roentgenographic and manometric methods were used.

3.3.1 Roentgenographic Observation

Contrast roentgenography of patients with perforated eardrums was carried out in the same manner as described above. Movement of the tube during repeated swallowing was filmed at a speed of 24 frames/s. Cineroentgenograms were analyzed frame by frame to determine the process of the pumping function of the tube. Two of nine cases are presented.

Patient 1. This patient was a 32-year-old man (Fig. 3.6). Frame a in Fig. 3.6 shows the tube closed at rest. Frames b–c show the shape of the tube during swallowing. The tubal lumen was dilated and filled with contrast medium. During this period, the contrast medium moved gradually to the distal side of the tube. Frame c corresponds to the final stage of swallowing. The contrast medium began to flow out of the tube along the tubal eminence. At the end of swallowing (frame d), most of the contrast medium flowed out as a result of closure of the tubal lumen.

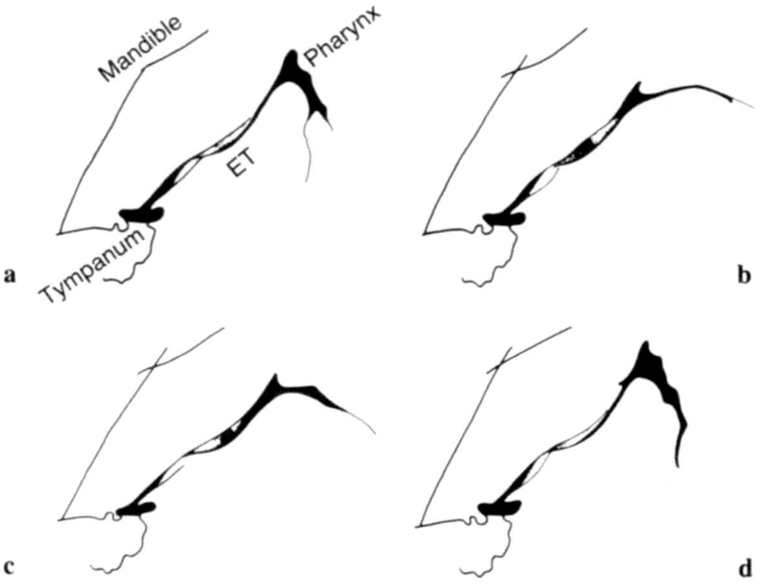

Fig. 3.6a–d. Cineroentgenograms of human eustachian tube in swallowing **a** Before swallowing; **b, c** during swallowing; **d** final stage of swallowing. Reproduced from Honjo et al (1981) Arch Otolaryngol 107:350–352. © 1981 American Medical Association

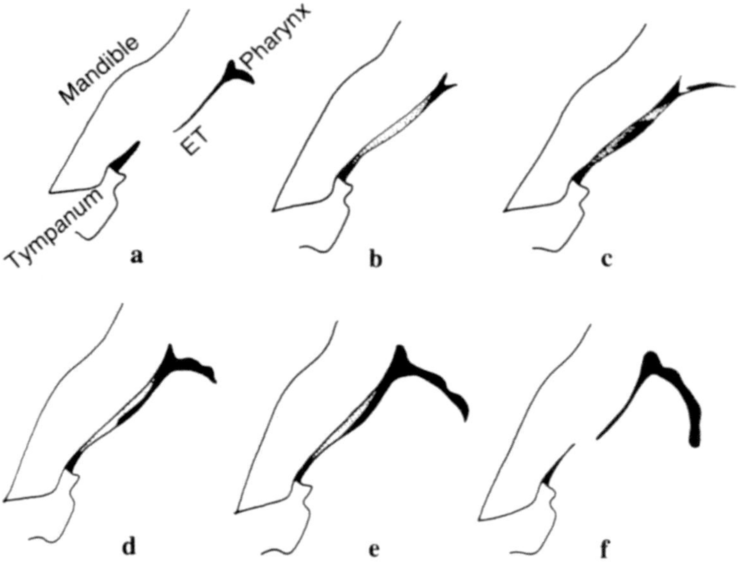

Fig. 3.7a–f. Pumplike discharge of fluid from tube. **a** Before, **b–d** during, **e** at final stage, and **f** after swallowing. Reproduced from Honjo et al (1981) Arch Otolaryngol 107:350–352. © 1981 American Medical Association

Patient 2. This patient was a 36-year-old man (Fig. 3.7). Frame a shows the closed tube at rest. During swallowing (frames b–d), the tube increased in diameter and became filled with the contrast medium; at the final stage of swallowing (frames e, f), the contrast medium flowed out to the pharynx, as observed in patient 1.

The present study clearly shows that the pumplike function of the tube consists of the accumulation of the fluid in the tube during tensor contraction and its discharge at the closing phase of tensor relaxation.

3.3.2 Mechanism of Muscular Clearance

To examine the mechanism of muscular clearance, the following two experiments were performed using cats, dogs, and monkeys.

3.3.2.1 Experiment 1

Tympanic pressure, including that in the eustachian tube, was measured when the tensor and levator muscles contracted. A small polyvinyl tube was connected to the middle ear through a hole made in the mastoid to measure the tympanic pressure. Bipolar hooked electrodes were inserted into the muscles from the oral side for electric stimulation. By the tensor stimulation, pressure in the middle ear slightly decreased, as shown in the upper part of Fig. 3.8. Stimulation of the levator, however, produced no decrease in the tympanic pressure.

Next, the pressure change during swallowing was examined. The tympanic pressure and the electromyogram (EMG) of the tensor, which indicated swal-

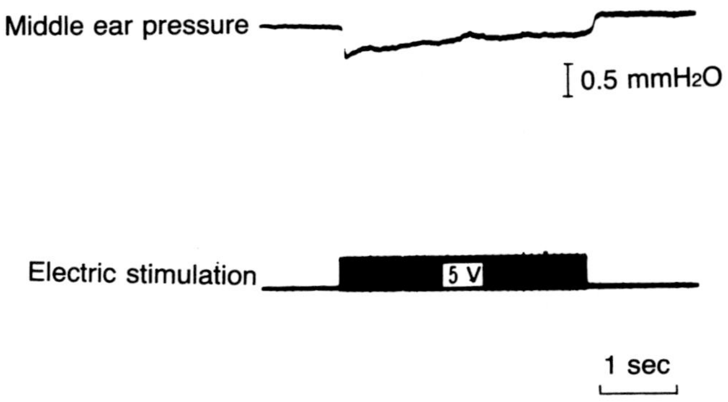

Fig. 3.8. Negative middle ear pressure during electric stimulation of tensor muscle

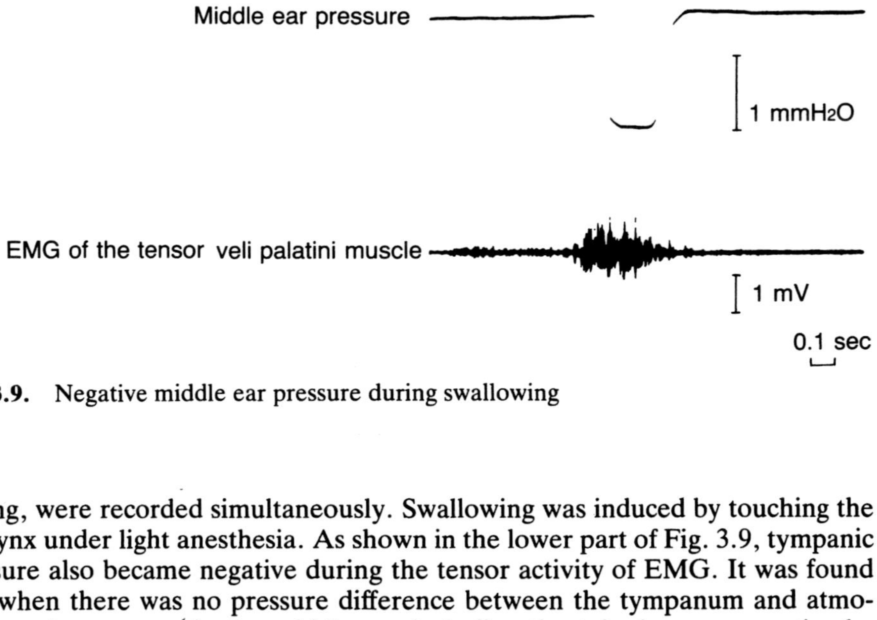

Fig. 3.9. Negative middle ear pressure during swallowing

lowing, were recorded simultaneously. Swallowing was induced by touching the pharynx under light anesthesia. As shown in the lower part of Fig. 3.9, tympanic pressure also became negative during the tensor activity of EMG. It was found that when there was no pressure difference between the tympanum and atmosphere, the pressure in the middle ear including the tube became negative by contraction of the tensor. This negative pressure is attributed to the dilatation of the tube, because the tympanic cavity is immobile. It appears that contraction of the tensor during swallowing enlarges the tubal lumen, resulting in the negative pressure.

3.3.2.2 Experiment 2

Movement of fluid through the tube by muscle contraction was observed in dogs and cats. Under general anesthesia, the tympanic bullae were removed for direct visualization of the tympanic cavity. Indigo carmine solution was instilled around the tympanic orifice of the tube. The pharyngeal orifice of the tube was observed with an endoscope through the palate. The tensor and levator muscles were stimulated electrically in the same manner described above.

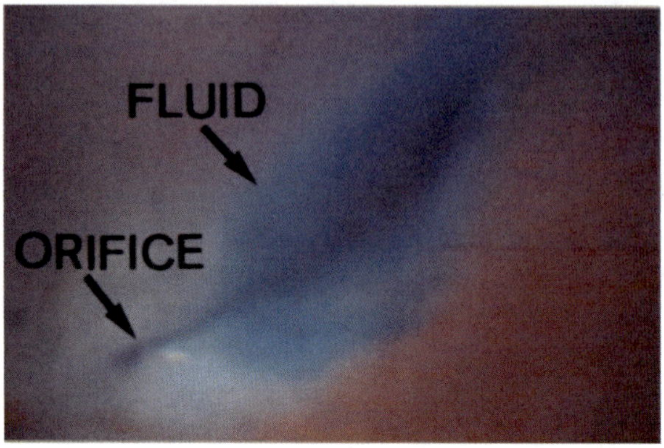

Fig. 3.10. Outflow of the fluid seen in pharyngeal orifice of eustachian tube

By electric stimulation of the tensor, colored fluid around the tympanic orifice was sucked into the tube. However, levator stimulation resulted in no movement of the fluid. In the pharyngeal orifice of the tube, periodic outflow of the solution was observed upon tensor stimulation (Fig. 3.10). More precisely, it flowed out of the orifice simultaneously with cessation of the stimulation. On the other hand, stimulation itself produced no outflow of the solution.

Thus, the sucking and discharging processes of the fluid through the tube were demonstrated as follows. First, negative pressure in the tube caused fluid in the tympanum to flow into the tube. Then, the fluid was held in the tube for a short time despite several muscle contractions. Then, the fluid that accumulated in the tube flowed out into the pharynx when the pressure in the tube increased by relaxation of the tensor muscle. Repeated dilatations and reductions of the tubal lumen make up the pumping function, which cleared large volumes of fluid from the middle ear into the pharynx.

3.4 Comparison of Clearance Function and Effects of Viscosity

Ciliary clearance of the tube also plays an important role in removal of fluid from the ear, though the amount is relatively small; conversely, muscular clearance causes massive discharge of fluid. The effects of viscosity of the fluid on these two activities and the quantitative difference between muscular and ciliary clearance were examined.

3.4.1 Effect of Viscosity on Ciliary Clearance

First, using various viscosities of fluid dye, elimination by ciliary activity was examined in cats. Under general anesthesia, the tensor muscle was severed to minimize muscular clearance. Colored fluid (0.02 ml) of various viscosities was introduced into the tympanum. To measure the interval between the instillation of the fluid and the beginning of its discharge from the orifice, the tubal orifice in the pharynx was observed by an endoscope.

The clearance time tended to increase with higher viscosities of the fluid, as

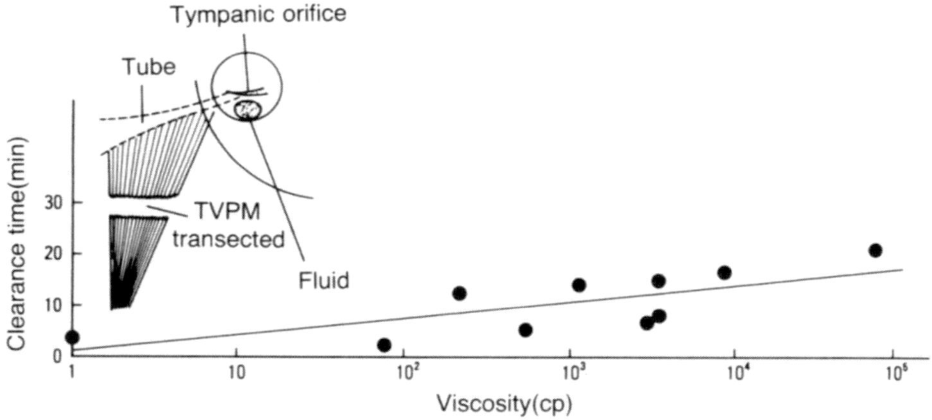

Fig. 3.11. Ciliary clearance function in relation to viscosity of fluid

Fig. 3.12. Test of muscular clearance of the tube by electric stimulation of tensor veli palatini muscle (*TVPM*)

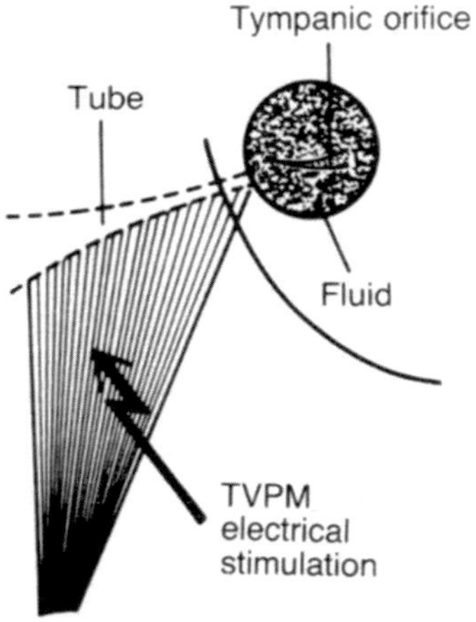

shown in Fig. 3.11. Although the time of passage of the dye through the eustachian tube increased with the viscosity of the fluid, fluids began to be discharged from the distal end of the tube within 15 min.

3.4.2 Effect of Viscosity on Muscular Clearance

Under general anesthesia, the tympanic cavity of the cat was filled with colored fluid of various viscosities, and the pharyngeal orifice of the tube was observed endoscopically. To simulate swallowing, the tensor muscle was electrically stimulated (Fig. 3.12). The number of contractions necessary for the massive discharge of fluid from the orifice was counted. When the fluid was not expelled by the muscle contractions, the interval between the instillation of the fluid and the beginning of its linear discharge by the ciliary clearance was measured.

Massive discharge was observed when the viscosity of the fluid was less than 570 cp. However, only a small amount of linear discharge was observed when

Table 3.2. Viscosity and muscular clearance function

Viscosity (cp[a])	Massive discharge[b]	Linear discharge
1	+, 1	−
80	+, 1	−
230	+, 1	−
570	+, 3	−
1,200	−	+
3,100	−	+
3,600	−	+
9,000	−	+
76,000	−	+

[a] Centipoise
[b] Numeral indicates number of muscular contractions needed for massive discharge

Table 3.3. Viscosity and muscle clearance function for fluid (0.02 ml) placed in the tympanum

Viscosity (cp[a])	Massive discharge	Linear discharge
80	−	+
1,200	−	+
3,100	−	+
3,600	−	+

[a] Centipoise

the viscosity was increased to more than 1200 cp (Table 3.2). It was revealed that massive discharge of fluid occurs in muscle contraction when the viscosity of the fluid is low. In contrast, only ciliary clearance occurs with highly viscous fluids.

On the other hand, when a small volume (0.02 ml) of fluid was introduced into the tympanum, no massive discharge was observed even after repeated electric stimulation of the muscle. It was found that when the volume of the fluid was small, it was removed only by ciliary clearance (Table 3.3).

The present study revealed two mechanisms of clearance in the eustachian tube. When the volume of fluid was large, clearance depended on the viscosity. Serous fluid was mainly cleared by muscular activity, while mucus was cleared both by ciliary and muscular activity.

3.4.3 Quantitative Comparison Between Muscular and Ciliary Clearance

It has been accepted that ciliary clearance is slow but continuous, while muscular clearance is intermittent but able to expel a larger volume of fluid. To evaluate the quantitative difference between ciliary and muscular clearance, experiments using colorimetry were carried out in cats. The tympanic bulla was filled with 0.4% indigo carmine under general anesthesia. The solution flowing out of the pharyngeal orifice of the tube was aspirated and measured quantita-

Fig. 3.13. Amount of fluid cleared by cillary and muscular activity

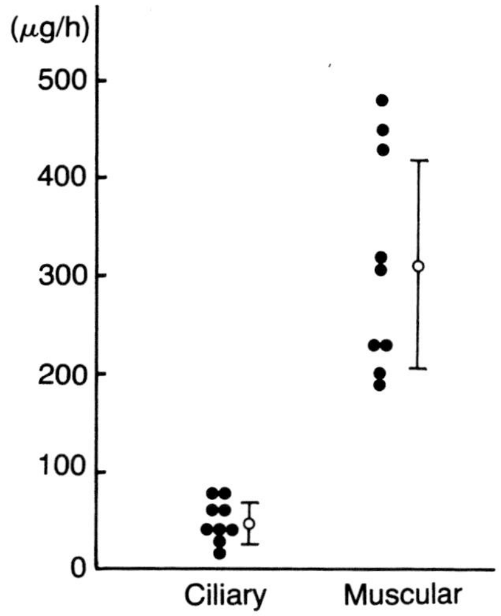

tively using a colorimeter. The amount of fluid discharged by ciliary activity was 49.4 ± 21 g/h, while it was 313.9 ± 106 g/h by muscular clearance, which is more than six times the amount with ciliary clearance (Fig. 3.13).

These results indicate that muscular clearance is more effective than ciliary clearance with fluids of low viscosity. The clearance of highly viscous fluid, however, is difficult without the assistance of ciliary clearance.

3.5 Summary of Chapter

Although the tensor and levator veli palatini muscles have been regarded as tubal muscles in opening the eustachian tube, the present observations revealed that the levator muscle had no effect on tubal function, except for dilation of the pharyngeal end of the tube. On the other hand, the tensor muscle was found to be the only muscle involved in opening the tube, by anterolateral pull of the tubal cartilage at the origin of the muscle.

Though ventilation of the middle ear appears to be the major function of the tube, clearance of the ear is also important when there is an accumulation of fluid, as seen in otitis media or after middle ear surgery. Two ways of tubal clearance have been proposed—ciliary and muscular clearance.

With regard to muscular clearance of the tube, repeated contractions and relaxations of the tensor during swallowing produced a pumplike action, which was six times more effective than ciliary clearance. However, it was also revealed that the relative importance of muscular and ciliary clearance varied with the condition of the middle ear fluid. In expelling low-viscosity fluids, massive fluid discharge by muscular clearance played the primary role, but as the viscosity increased ciliary clearance became important. Thus, the combined action of muscular and ciliary clearance contributes to effective drainage of fluids from the middle ear.

References

Aschan G (1955) The anatomy of the eustachian tube with regard to its function. Acta Soc Med Upsal 60:131–149

Cantekin EI, Doyle WJ, Reichert T, Phillips BA, Bluestone CD (1979) Dilation of the eustachian tube by electrical stimulation of the mandibular nerve. Ann Otol Rhinol Laryngol 88:40–51

Holborow CA (1962) Deafness associated with cleft palate. J Laryngol Otol 76:762–773

Honjo I, Ushiro K, Okazaki N, Kumazawa T (1981) Evaluation of eustachian tube function by contrast roentgenography. Arch Otolaryngol 107:350–352

McMyn JK (1940) The anatomy of the salpingo-pharyngeus muscle. J Laryngol Otol 55:1–22

Politzer (1909) Diseases of the ear. Lea and Febiger, Philadelphia

Rich AR (1920) A physiological study of the eustachian tube and its related muscles. Johns Hopkins Bull 31:206–214

Toynbee J (1853) On the muscle which opens the eustachian tube. Proc Roy Soc London 6:286–287

Zöllner F (1942) Anatomie, Physiologie, Pathologie und Klinik der Ohrtrompete und ihrer diagnostisch therapeutischen Beziehungen zu allen Nachbarschaftserkrankungen. Springer, Berlin

Chapter 4
Evaluation of Static and Dynamic Functions of Eustachian Tube

Since the eustachian tube has two functions—ventilation of the middle ear and clearance of foreign bodies from the ear, tests for tubal function are divided into two groups—aerodynamic tests for ventilatory function and clearance tests.

Evaluation of the tubal functions with these methods, however, becomes rather difficult when the tympanic membrane is intact or any fluid is present in the middle ear (Fig. 4.1). In the studies presented here, therefore, all the tests were performed in ears with perforated eardrums after the removal of the ear fluid. Since myringotomy is a routine procedure for the treatment of otitis media with effusion (OME), perforations made for the treatment were utilized. In chronic otitis media, examinations were made through already existing tympanic perforations. Myringotomy was performed only in patients with cholesteatoma who had intact eardrums, with informed consent of patients.

In addition to the conventional tests for eustachian tube function, new tests such as phototubometry, which is a method of light-mediated evaluation of tubal opening, manosonotubometry, which assesses tubal opening and closing by sound and air pressure, and flowmetry, which measures tubal compliance by constant air flow through the tube, were developed or modified in this study. For comprehensive evaluation of the eustachian tube with ear diseases such as

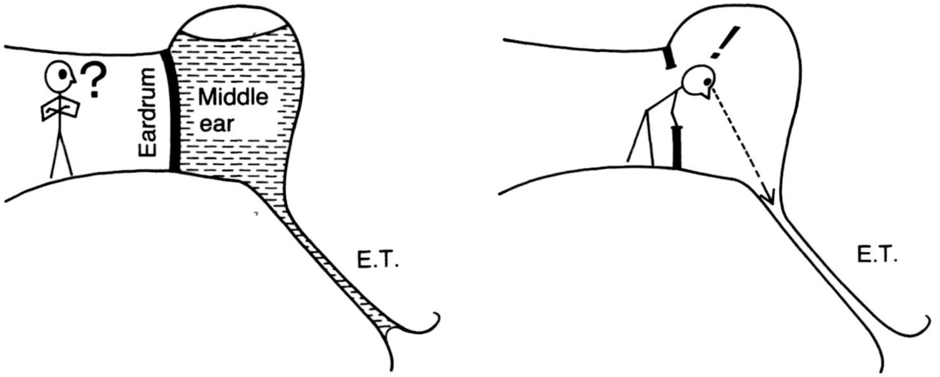

Fig. 4.1. Advantage of eardrum perforation for evaluation of tubal function. *E.T.* eustachian tube

OME, chronic otitis media, or cholesteatoma, these tests were performed on the same patients in subsequent chapters. The method of examination, the normal range for each test, and advantages and disadvantages of the tests are described below.

4.1 Conventional Tests for Ventilatory and Clearance Functions of Eustachian Tube

4.1.1 Examination of Ventilatory Function of Eustachian Tube

Since the eustachian tube is closed at rest and opens only momentarily during swallowing, the ventilatory function of the tube has to be evaluated under both conditions. The examinations for this function were divided into two: the degree of tubal closure at rest (static condition) and the degree of its opening during swallowing (dynamic condition).

4.1.1.1 Test for Static Condition of Eustachian Tube

Air pressure was applied to the middle ear through the tympanic perforation, and the minimum pressure necessary for spontaneous opening of the tube was determined. Previous investigators have applied middle ear pressures of up to 400 mmH_2O. However, as some patients with stenosis of the tube needed a greater pressure, we applied up to 800 mmH_2O in this study. The tube was judged to have stenosis or obstruction when it did not open even at this pressure.

After making the ear canal airtight, the middle ear pressure was increased until there was a sudden drop in the pressure due to opening of the tube. These pressure changes were recorded with a pressure transducer (Fig. 4.2). In the normal ear, the minimum pressure for static condition of the tube was usually the same even with repeated testing (Fig. 4.3).

In 33 normal ears (23 adults and 10 children with traumatic tympanic perforation), the minimum pressure for opening the tube was determined. The mean value of the pressure was 355 mmH_2O and, with two standard deviations, 165–

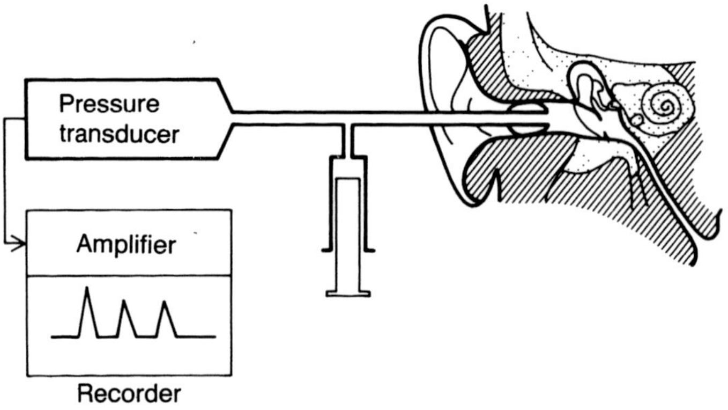

Fig. 4.2. Test system for ventilation function of eustachian tube

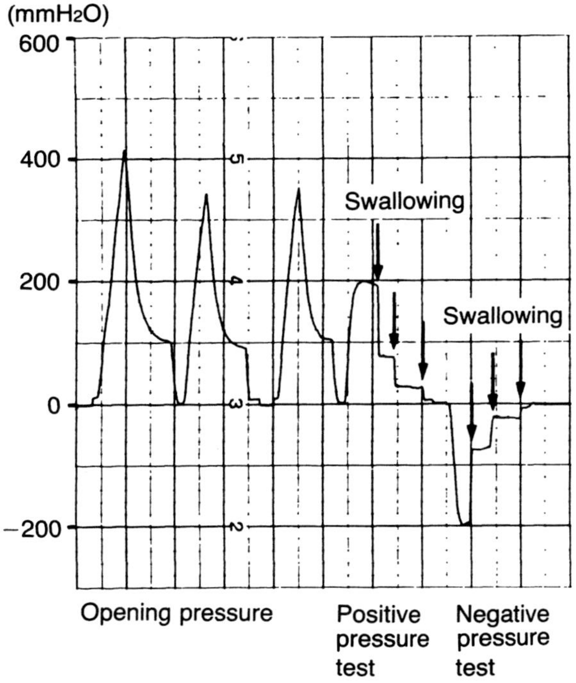

Fig. 4.3. Wave form in normal ear (static and dynamic tubal function tests)

545 mmH_2O was regarded to be the normal range for the opening pressure under static condition of the tube (Fig. 4.4). This value was similar to that reported by Yuasa and Takakura (28 ± 15.5 mmHg) and Bluestone and Cantekin (1981; 330 mmH_2O) and roughly agreed with a mean of 3.86 kPa in children and 4.19 kPa in adults reported by Bylander (1980).

4.1.1.2 Test for Dynamic Condition of Eustachian Tube

This test examines the degree of tubal opening after swallowing. Since the first reports by Flisberg et al. (1963) and Miller (1965), the test has been widely used as a dynamic test for the ventilatory function of the tube. Although the positive or negative pressure applied to the middle ear varies among different investigators, it was set at ±200 mmH_2O in the present study. The dynamic function in the tube was assessed by the decrease of applied pressure to atmospheric pressure after swallowings (Fig. 4.3). The criteria for normal ears in this test had previously not been well established. Using 33 ears with traumatic perforation of the eardrum, the normal range for the test was determined in the present study.

Positive pressure applied to the middle ear could be reduced to atmospheric pressure in 24 (72.7%) of the 33 ears, and to less than 50% in all the ears. Therefore, the normal range for the positive pressure test was considered to be the reduction of the applied pressure to a level of less than 50% (Fig. 4.5).

When negative pressure was applied to the middle ear, however, only 29 (84.8%) of 33 ears could reduce the pressure to less than 50%, suggesting that this range is not appropriate as a criterion for the normal ear. Since 96.9% of the ears could reduce the applied pressure of −200 mmH_2O to some extent by swallowing, ears that showed a decrease in negative pressure toward atmospheric

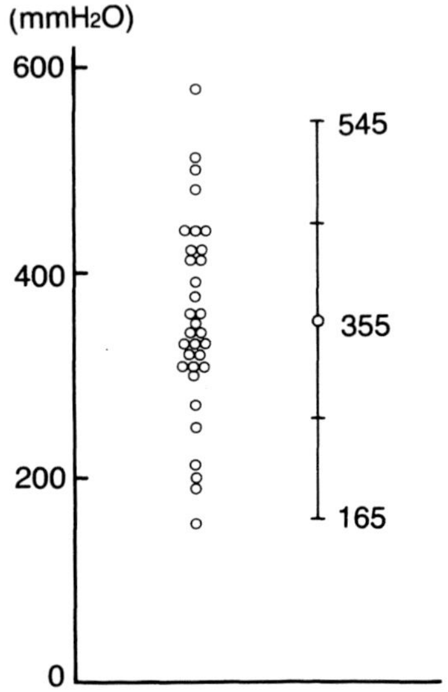

Fig. 4.4. Normal range of tubal opening pressure based on 33 normal ears (means ± 2 SD)

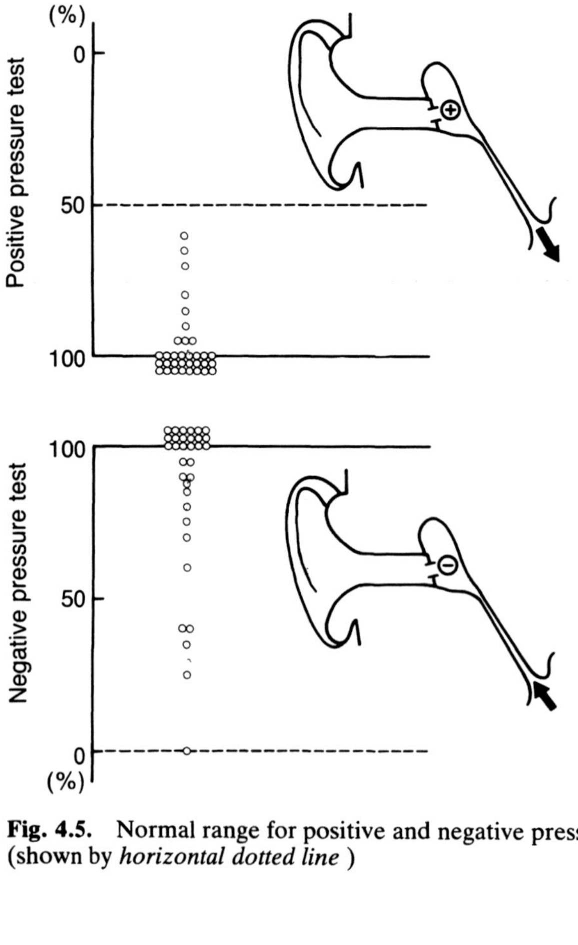

Fig. 4.5. Normal range for positive and negative pressure tests based on 33 normal ears (shown by *horizontal dotted line*)

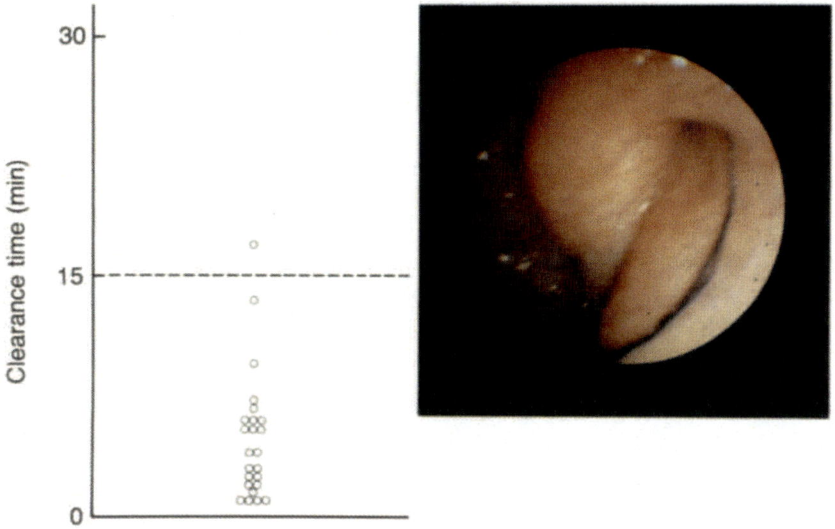

Fig. 4.6. Normal range of time for dye solution clearance based on 24 normal ears (shown by *horizontal dotted line*). *Inset* shows solution expelled from pharyngeal orifice of tube

pressure were regarded as normal in this test. Bylander (1980) reported that 53% of children's ears and 9% of adults' ears were incapable of reducing negative pressures. The discrepancy between these results and ours is considered to be due to differences in the conditions of evaluation (with a perforated eardrum at a pressure of -200 mmH_2O). In the following study, the present data from 33 normal controls were used as reference values for dynamic function of the perforated ears.

4.1.2 Examination of Clearance Function of Eustachian Tube

When any fluid is retained in the middle ear cavity, the eustachian tube begins to drain it into the nasopharynx. This drainage function can also be divided into the static component (ciliary clearance), involving continuous discharge of a small amount at rest, and the dynamic component (muscular clearance), which is characterized by a massive and intermittent discharge by swallowing. Since quantitative evaluation of the dynamic component is rather difficult, the static component was examined in this study. Although a number of methods have been developed here, we used a simple test in which a small amount (0.02 cm^3) of dye solution (0.4% indigo carmine) was introduced into the middle ear through the perforation. The time for the solution to be expelled from the pharyngeal orifice was measured by transnasal endoscopy (Fig. 4.6). Observation was made for a maximum of 30 min.

As discharge of the dye was within 15 min in 23 (95.8%) of the 24 normal ears examined, 15 min was considered to be the normal range for clearance of the eustachian tube (Fig. 4.6).

4.2 Phototubometry and Sonotubometry

A method to evaluate dynamic function of the eustachian tube was developed using light. On the other hand, sonotubometry has been improved by many investigators since the reports by Dishoek (1937) and Perlman (1939). In the present study, by adding the pressure component to sonotubometry, an improvement of the sound test was attempted.

4.2.1 Phototubometry

In this test, a fiberscope (ENF-P, Olympus, Tokyo, Japan), as light source, was placed at the pharyngeal orifice of the tube through the nose. The light reaching the eardrum through the eustachian tube was detected by a highly sensitive silicon diode (S874-18C, Hamamatsu Photonics, Hamamatsu, Japan), which was placed in the ear canal when the tube opened during swallowing (Fig. 4.7).

The fiberscopic images were monitored on a television screen to examine the movements of the pharyngeal orifice of the tube. Light signals detected in the ear canal were superimposed by a videogram (VG-40, FORA, Osaka, Japan) over the endoscopic view of the tube. The amount of information increased markedly when this examination was combined with sonotubometry, which is described in the following.

Figure 4.8 shows a simultaneous recording of the endoscopic image of the pharyngeal orifice, a phototubometric wave, and a sonotubometric wave. The photo- and sonotubometric waves showed a sudden rise at the opening of the

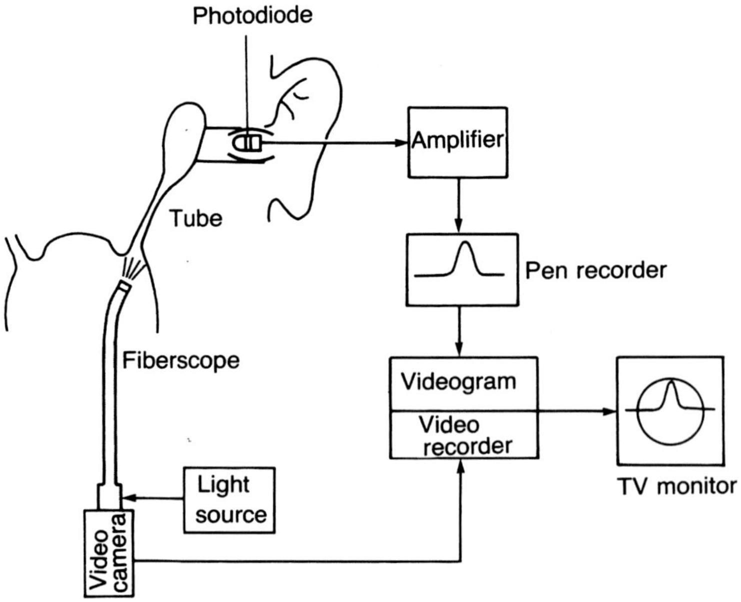

Fig. 4.7. System of "phototubometry"

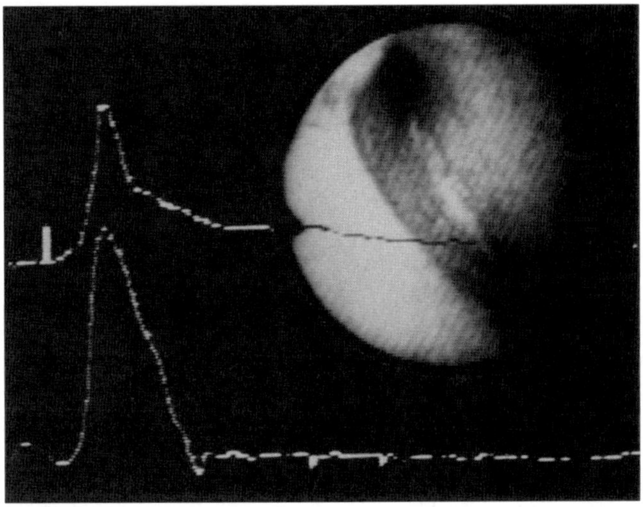

Fig. 4.8. Simultaneous recording of endoscopic image of pharyngeal orifice, phototubometric wave, and sonotubometric wave

pharyngeal orifice during swallowing, indicating that not just the pharyngeal orifice but the entire length of the eustachian tube opens at this moment.

Normal phototubometric waves are presented in Fig. 4.9. A simultaneous recording of sonotubometric waves is shown at the bottom of each wave. Figure 4.9a is an example of the most frequent type of monophasic pattern, and Fig. 4.9b is a pattern with a gently falling phase. Two-peak waves (Fig. 4.9c) and biphasic waves (Fig. 4.9d) were also observed. The time-lag between the peaks of photo- and sonotubometric waves is considered to be due to the faster transmission of light than sound. An advantage of phototubometry is that it indicates the exact moment and duration of tubal opening simultaneously with the endoscopic information around the pharyngeal end of the tube.

4.2.2 Manosonotubometry

The principle of the sonometric method is that the sound introduced into the nasopharynx from the nose is picked up in the external ear canal. Thus, the extent of the tubal opening can be assessed by the increase in sound intensity during swallowing. Though this method has improved markedly since that originally performed, accurate evaluation of tubal function may still be difficult when the ear has a thickened drum or contains fluid. Therefore, in the present study, the test was carried out in ears with a perforated drum. At the same time as the sonotubometric test, manometric evaluation of the tube was made by applying pressure to the middle ear via the perforation.

A small microphone (ET-20, Rion, Tokyo, Japan) and a pressure transducer (P3000S-501D-02, Copal, Tokyo, Japan) were placed in the ear canal in an airtight fashion, and a syringe to supply pressure to the middle ear was connected to this system. FM sound at 5–9 kHz (modulated to 660 Hz), with a sound

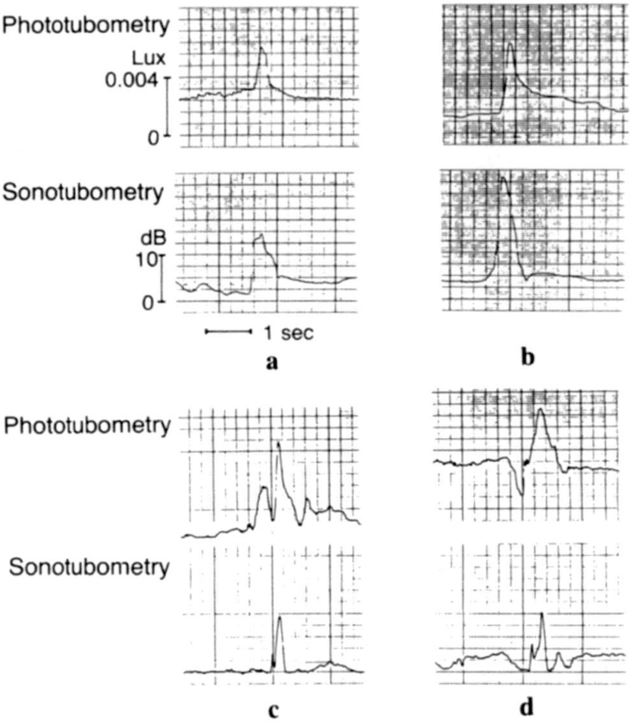

Fig. 4.9a–d. Normal wave forms obtained by phototubometry and sonotubometry

pressure level of 120 dB, was introduced into the nasopharynx via the nostril. The sound detected in the ear canal was recorded after decibel conversion (Fig. 4.10).

4.2.2.1 Normal Eustachian Tube

As shown in Fig. 4.11, the sound pressure picked up in the ear canal increased for a short time when the tube was opened by an increase in the middle ear pressure. The negative pressure returned to atmospheric pressure with the opening sign of swallowing in the sonometric wave, suggesting normal function of the tube.

4.2.2.2 Closing Failure of Eustachian Tube

Since this examination permitted objective evaluation of closing failure of the tube, representative cases are described in the following.

Patient 1. The patient was a 57-year-old man with OME. In this patient, the sound pressure of the ear canal began to increase as the middle ear pressure reached 30 mmH_2O, indicating enlargement of the tubal cavity at a relatively low pressure of the middle ear (Fig. 4.12). Then, the sound wave suddenly increased, indicating opening of the eustachian tube at an ear pressure of 180 mmH_2O. After that, the pressure in the ear decreased to the original level, while

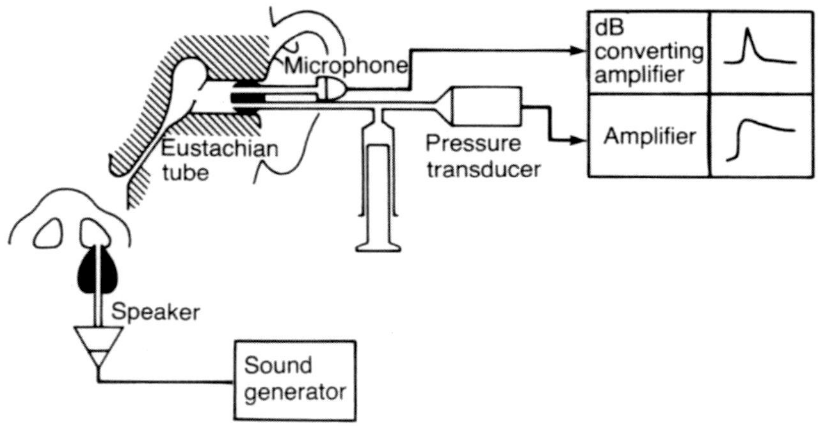

Fig. 4.10. System of "manosonotubometry"

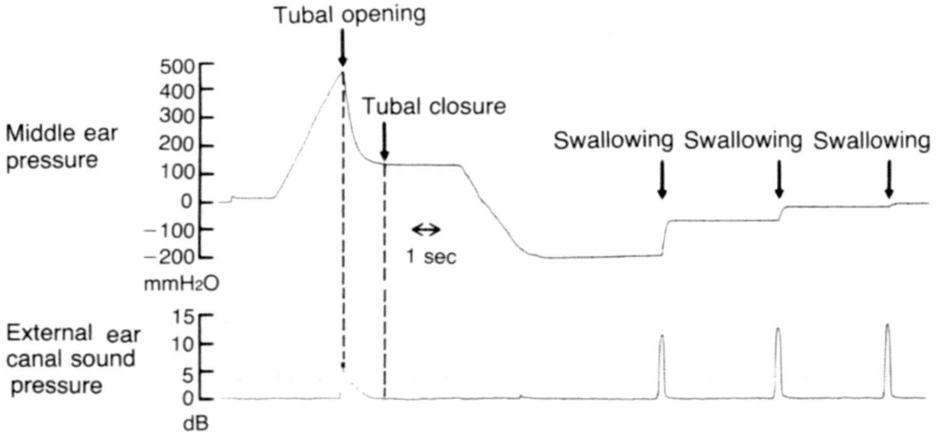

Fig. 4.11. Normal wave form obtained by manosonotubometry

the sound level remained elevated, suggesting incomplete closure of the tube. By applying negative middle ear pressure, the sound level returned for the first time to the original level by complete closure of the tube. As this patient could not reduce negative middle ear pressure by swallowing, he was judged also to have opening failure of the tube.

Bluestone and Cantekin (1981) reported a "floppy tube," which was easily locked by negative middle ear pressure, despite low pressure for opening the tube. The present study demonstrated such a condition of "floppy tube" in the characteristic waves of the sound and air pressure.

Patient 2. The patient was a 33-year-old man with OME. In this patient, a negative middle ear pressure of −200 mmH_2O was equalized by swallowing, which indicated normal opening function of the tube (Fig. 4.13). However, the

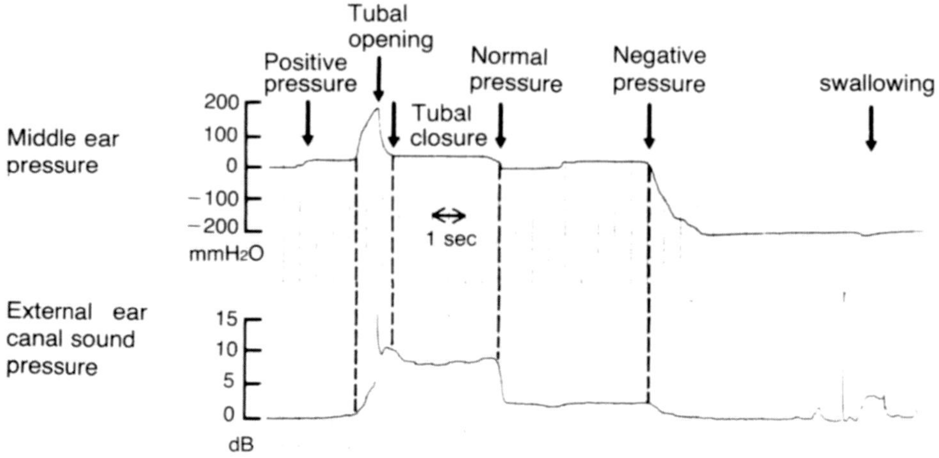

Fig. 4.12. Wave form in a patient with closing failure of tube

sound level in the ear canal remained elevated even after swallowing, suggesting disturbance of the tube in closing. When the patient was asked to sniff, the sound level decreased to the original level simultaneously with the formation of negative pressure in the ear. It was suggested that the eustachian tube of this patient was closed by the negative pressure due to sniffing.

Magnuson (1978) and Magnuson and Falk (1983) termed such a pathological condition of the tube in which negative middle ear pressure develops by sniffing "closing failure of the tube." This manosonotubometric test clearly demonstrated not only the closing failure of the tube, but also the development of negative middle ear pressure by sniffing, with the resultant closure of the tube.

Manosonotubometry was found to be useful, especially in the detection of closing failure of the tube, because it allows evaluation of both the opening and closing processes of the tube by the pressure component added to this test.

4.2.3 Flowmetry

Examinations of the eustachian tube, including the methods described above, were not suitable for measuring the capacity of the tube to open. The degree of tubal patency, excluding factors such as the fluid in the tube, has also proved impossible to examine with conventional tests. The forced response test (FRT) developed by Cantekin et al. (1977) examines both patency of the eustachian tube itself and its dynamic opening function by applying a constant air flow through the tube.

By continuous recording of the tubal resistance, assessment of the dynamic condition of the eustachian tube during swallowing was made possible. Compliance of the tube, which has been difficult to determine objectively, could also be evaluated by obtaining the ratio of resistance when the flow rate through the tube changed.

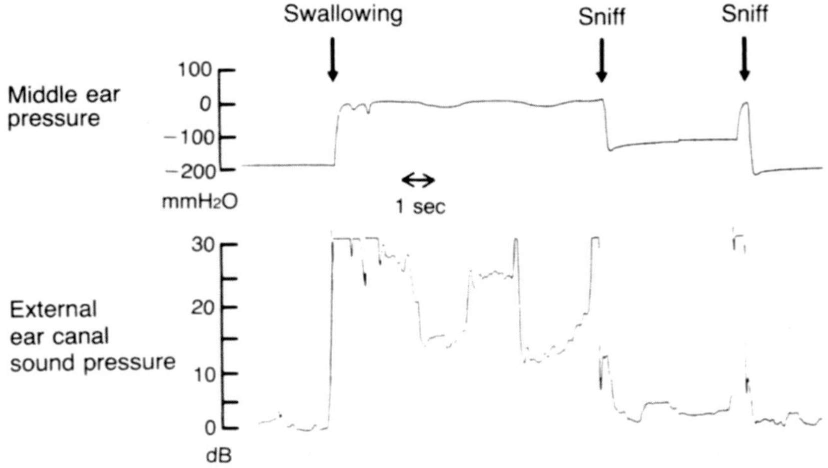

Fig. 4.13. Negative middle ear pressure produced by sniffing in patient with incomplete closure of tube

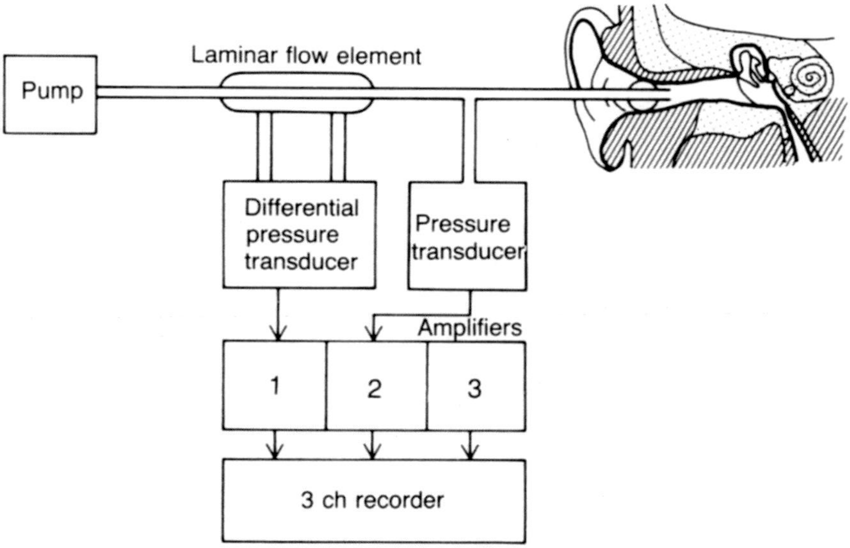

Fig. 4.14. System used for tubal resistance test

4.2.3.1 Methods of Evaluation

In ears with perforated drums, constant air flow was introduced into the middle ear with a pump system. The pressure of air applied to the middle ear was increased until the eustachian tube opened. By maintaining the air flow at a constant rate, the flow rate and pressure were simultaneously recorded while the tube was kept open. The resistance of the tube was continuously calculated and recorded by a multiplication-division amplifier (Fig. 4.14).

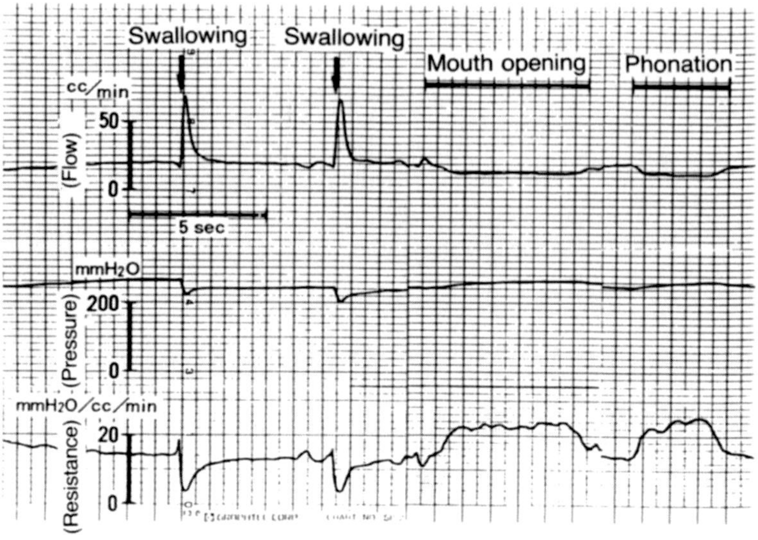

Fig. 4.15. Normal wave forms in tubal resistance test

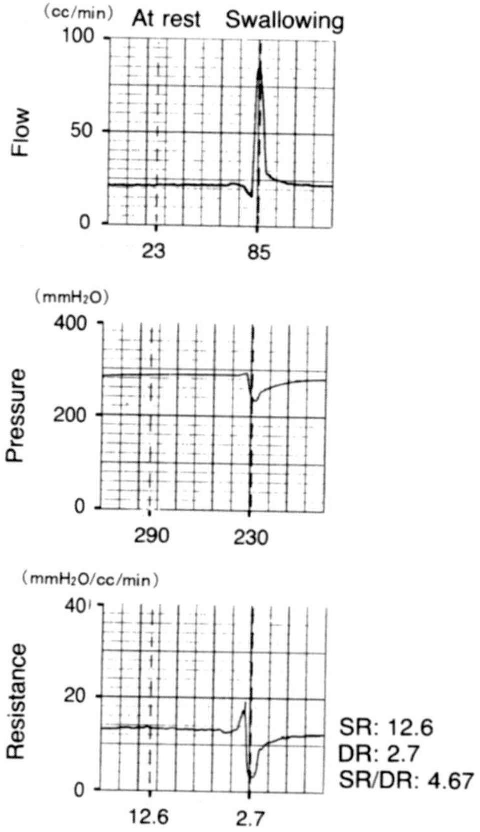

Fig. 4.16. Method for calculating force required to open tube during swallowing. *SR* static resistance, *DR* dynamic resistance

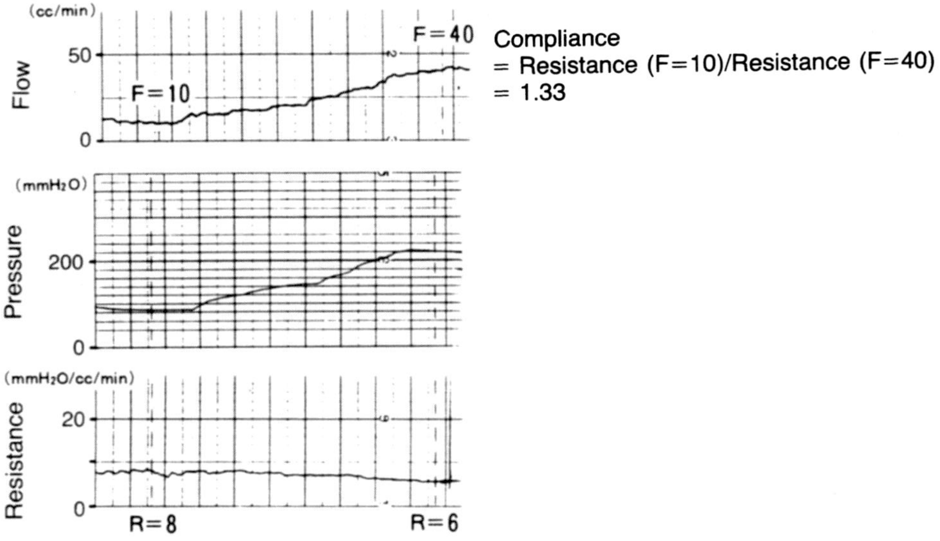

Fig. 4.17. Measurement of compliance of eustachian tube by changing flow rate through tube

In this study, the resistance of the eustachian tube at a flow rate of 20 cm^3/min was determined as the static resistance (SR) of the tube. The resistance during swallowing was regarded as the dynamic resistance (DR) of the tube. Normal ears (traumatic tympanic perforation) showed a reduction in the resistance during swallowing, indicating opening of the tube (Fig. 4.15). SR/DR was considered to represent the dynamic force of the tube in opening. Figure 4.16 shows the method used to calculate the opening force of the tube from the reduction in resistance during swallowing. This value is 1 or more in the normal eustachian tube.

4.2.3.2 Compliance of Eustachian Tube

The compliance of the eustachian tube was determined by changing the flow rate through the tube. The resistance of the tube decreased as the flow rate increased, because of increase in diameter of the tube (Fig. 4.17). Thus, the ability of the tube to dilate or compliance of the tube can be evaluated by the ratio of the resistance at 10 and 40 cm^3/min. The normal ratio for the compliance of the tube was considered to be 1.80 ($\pm$0.47):1 in this study.

Thus, flowmetry permits both quantitative evaluation of the opening force of the tube and determination of the tubal compliance.

4.3 Summary of Chapter

The normal range of eustachian tube function in both ventilatory and clearance functions was established in normal subjects with traumatic perforation of the eardrum. In addition to conventional tests of the tube, the validity of new tests, such as phototubometry, manosonotubometry for examination of closing failure, and flowmetry for measurement of both resistance and compliance of the tube, was confirmed.

References

Bluestone CD, Cantekin EI (1981) Panel on experiences with testing eustachian tube function. Current clinical methods, indications and interpretation of eustachian tube function tests. Ann Otol Rhinol Laryngol 90:552–562

Bylander A (1980) Comparison of eustachian tube function in children and adults with normal ear. Ann Otol Rhinol Laryngol 89 (Suppl 68):20–24

Cantekin EI, Bluestone CD, Saez CA, Doyle WJ, Philips DC (1977) Normal and abnormal middle ear ventilation. Ann Otol Rhinol Laryngol 86 (Suppl 41):1–15

Dishoek HAEv (1937) Das Pneumophon. Arch Ohr Nase Kehlkopfheilkunde 144:53–58

Flisberg K, Ingelstedt S, Örtegren U (1963) Controlled ear aspiration of air. A physiological test of the tubal function. Acta Otolaryngol Suppl 182:35–38

Magnuson B (1978) Tubal closing failure in retraction type cholesteatoma and adhesive middle ear lesions. Acta Otolaryngol 86:408–417

Magnuson B, Falk B (1983) Eustachian tube malfunction and middle ear disease in new prospective. J Otolaryngol 12:187–193

Miller GF (1965) Eustachian tubal function in normal and diseased ears. Arch Otolaryngol 81:41–48

Perlman HB (1939) The eustachian tube. Abnormal patency and normal physiologic state. Arch Otolaryngol 30:212–238

Yuasa R, Takakura M (1971) Analysis of physical properties of the eustachian tube. J Otolaryngol Jpn 74:749–754 (in Japanese)

Chapter 5
Otitis Media with Effusion and Eustachian Tube

The close relation between otitis media with effusion (OME) and the eustachian tube has been widely accepted, as indicated by the term "catarrh of the eustachian tube" used almost synonymously with OME. One of the reasons for such a view is based on the accumulated clinical experience that the patency of the eustachian tube as determined by tubal inflation is impaired in most OME patients. This view is also supported by the frequent occurrence of OME in patients with nasopharyngeal carcinoma or hypertrophic adenoid, which may cause stenosis of the eustachian tube, and by animal experiments in which middle ear effusion was induced by ligating the tube. However, in the pathogenesis of OME with respect to eustachian tube dysfunction, we have as yet no explanation except for the "hydrops ex vacuo" theory (primary eustachian tube obstruction producing effusion in the middle ear).

On the other hand, studies have demonstrated the presence of bacteria (Senturia et al. 1958; Kokko 1974; Liu et al. 1975) and endotoxins (Bernstein et al. 1980) in the effusion, and OME has been produced in animals by introducing immune complexes into the ear. These findings strongly suggest that inflammation plays an important role in the pathogenesis of OME. However, since the focus of this chapter is not inflammation but the eustachian tube in the development of OME, detailed reference to inflammation will be avoided.

One of the causes of difficulty in understanding the pathological condition of the eustachian tube in OME is the presence of secondary factors resulting from the disease, such as swelling of the mucous membrane in the tube or the retention of mucous fluid. These factors may obscure whether the impaired function of the tube is the cause or result of the disease. In the studies presented in this chapter, therefore, the eustachian tube was examined by several methods to clarify other factors that may affect OME, and tubal function was examined not only in the active stage of OME but also in its convalescent stage to estimate the initial condition of the tube.

Current problems concerning the relation between the eustachian tube and OME are: (a) Is there stenosis or obstruction of the eustachian tube in patients with OME? (b) what are the characteristic features of the eustachian tube in OME? and (c) how can the development of OME be explained with respect to eustachian tube dysfunction?

In addition, factors other than the eustachian tube that are necessary for the development and prolongation of OME will be discussed.

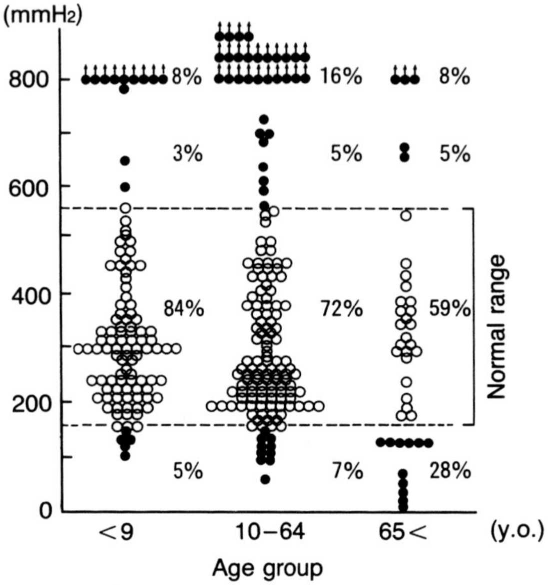

Fig. 5.1. Opening pressure of tube in 300 ears with OME

5.1 Eustachian Tube Function in OME

To obtain basic data concerning the extent and type of tubal dysfunction in OME, patients in the active stage of the disease were examined first. As the eardrum and effusion hinder examination of the tube, all subjects in this study were examined after myringotmomy and removal of the fluid by aspiration.

There have already been a number of reports on the function of the eustachian tube in OME (Silverstein et al. 1966; Bluestone et al. 1972; Holmquist and Renwall 1974; Cantekin et al. 1976), but only Bluestone et al. (1972) simultaneously evaluated the two functions of the tube, namely ventilation and clearance. In the present study, both functions were examined in 300 ears with OME. The subjects were divided into three groups according to age: 108 ears of children (4–9 years old), 153 ears of adolescents or adults (10–64 years old), and 39 ears of patients over 65 years old. The resistance of the tube was also measured by flowmetry for comparison with data obtained by conventional tests.

5.1.1 Is the Eustachian Tube Stenotic in OME?

First, the opening pressure of the eustachian tube was measured by applying positive pressure of up to 800 mmH_2O to the ear through the perforated eardrum. It was revealed that, contrary to our expectations, 75% of OME patients showed normal opening pressure of the tube, with a slight difference among the three groups (Fig. 5.1), while stenosis of the tube was noted only in 12%. In children, 84% of the ears were within the normal range of opening pressure, and only 8% showed stenosis of the eustachian tube. Cantekin et al. (1976) reported that the mean opening pressure in OME children was slightly higher than that in

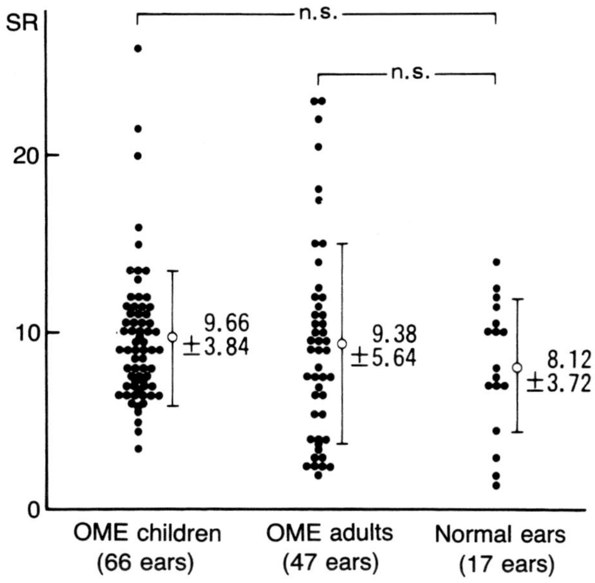

Fig. 5.2. Tubal resistance in OME patients and normal controls. *n.s.* not significant

normal children. The present findings coincide well with their results. On the other hand, 28% of the older patients showed low opening pressure of the tube, indicating a condition similar to a patulous eustachian tube.

Resistance of the eustachian tube was examined by flowmetry in 113 patients (66 children and 47 adults) with OME. Flowmetry by constant air flow through the tube allows assessment of the patency of the tube, excluding secondary factors such as viscous fluid in the tube. It was found that the tubal resistance in OME patients was not different from that of normal ears in both children and adults (Fig. 5.2). These results, together with the findings of opening pressure, indicate that organic stenosis of the tube is quite rare in OME patients.

It has long been believed that patients with OME have tubal stenosis in various degrees. Such misunderstanding has partly been due to viscous fluid obstructing the tube, which was judged to be stenotic by Politzer's maneuver or inflation by a catheter. Stenosis of the eustachian tube as a result of OME might be taken to be an etiological factor of the disease.

5.1.2 Does the Eustachian Tube in OME Open During Swallowing?

The eustachian tube in OME patients, even if not stenotic as revealed in the present study, may not open during swallowing, which is the most important function of the tube. Therefore, the dynamic function of the tube in relieving applied middle ear pressure by swallowing was examined in 290 ears of OME patients (Fig. 5.3).

The results of the positive pressure test were poor in 69% of the patients, suggesting that the tube does not easily open by swallowing even when there is no tubal obstruction at rest. However, this functional obstruction of the tube may again be a result of OME. To eliminate the confounding factors, static

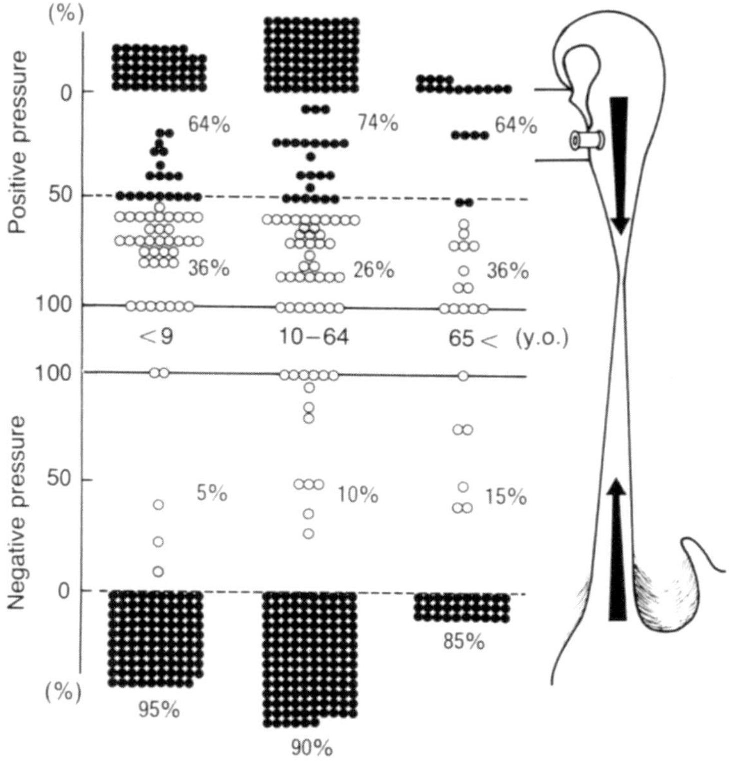

Fig. 5.3. Dynamic function of tube in 290 patients with OME

resistance (SR) of the tube at rest and dynamic resistance (DR) during swallowing were measured by flowmetry in 113 ears of OME patients (66 children and 47 adults; Fig. 5.4). The ratio of SR to DR obtained by flowmetry must be 1:1 or greater for dynamic opening of the tube during swallowing. The results were that in 35% of the children and in 40% of the adults the tube did not open even during swallowing. These results reveal that the dynamic function of the tube is impaired in OME and that this kind of tubal impairment is not necessarily a result of the disease.

The results of the negative pressure test showed a significant impairment of the tube. Ninety-one percent of the ears tested (95% in children) were incapable of relieving the negative middle ear pressure by swallowing. This finding was consistent with earlier reports (Silverstein et al. 1966; Westergaard 1970; Bluestone et al. 1972; Holmquist and Renwall 1974) and was considered to be characteristic of eustachian tube dysfunction in OME patients.

Considering the ability of the eustachian tube to relieve positive middle ear pressure, but not negative pressure, the eustachian tube in OME patients appears to act as a one-way valve that allows air to flow from the ear to the pharynx. The location of this valvelike structure in the tube was examined in ten adult patients with OME. Negative pressure (-200 mmH_2O) was applied to the

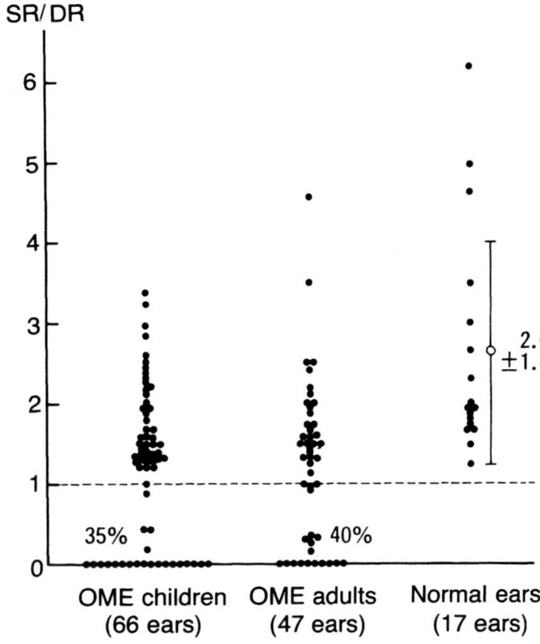

Fig. 5.4. Force to open tube during swallowing obtained by flowmetry *SR* static resistance, *DR* dynamic resistance

middle ear through the tympanic perforation and a polyethylene tube was advanced from the pharyngeal orifice into the eustachian tube during repeated swallowing. The point where the negative pressure was relieved by swallowing was judged to be the site of ventilatory dysfunction in the tube. This site was generally at the distal part of the tube, lower than the origin of the tensor muscle from the tubal cartilage (Fig. 5.5). This characteristic one-way valve action of the eustachian tube was considered to provide a clue to the pathogenesis of OME.

5.1.3 Clearance Function of Eustachian Tube

The ability of the tube to drain dye introduced into the middle ear through the perforation was examined in 230 ears with OME (Fig. 5.6). In 47% of ears examined, the dye was cleared from the pharyngeal orifice within the normal range of 15 min, while the discharge was delayed in the remaining 53%. This function was impaired in 62% of the OME children.

The present results suggest that the ciliary function of the eustachian tube is considerably impaired in the active stage of OME. However, whether this impairment is an essential pathological feature of OME or a condition secondary to the disease has not yet been determined. This will be referred to in Sect. 5.2.

5.1.4 Summary

The findings on the opening pressure, dynamic ventilatory function, and clearance function of the tube in 300 OME ears were as follows:

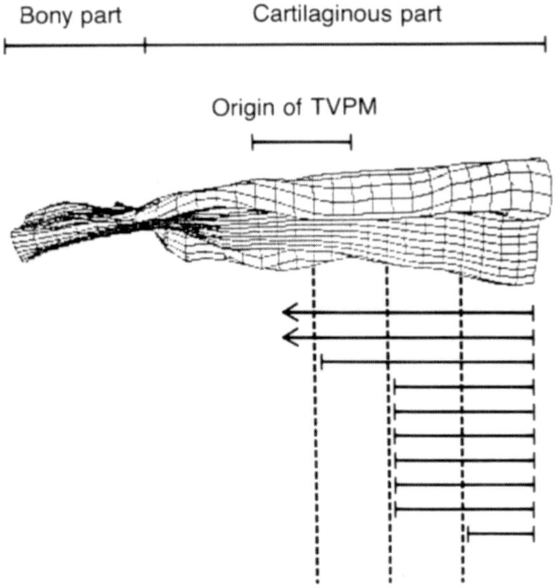

Fig. 5.5. Sites of disturbance for dynamic function of tube in ten ears with OME

a) Organic stenosis of the tube was uncommon, and it was unlikely that stenosis of the tube was the cause of OME.
b) The dynamic function of the tube in relieving negative pressure by swallowing was markedly impaired, suggesting that the tube acts as a one-way valve that permits air flow only from the middle ear to the pharynx.
c) The clearance function of the tube was impaired in about half of the ears examined.

5.2 Eustachian Tube in Convalescent Stage of OME

The OME patients we encounter in daily practice have a eustachian tube that is affected by secondary factors such as mucosal lesions or viscous fluid in the tube. Some studies have regarded these secondary factors as being characteristic of the eustachian tube in OME. Examination of the very early stage of OME or its convalescent stage after disappearance of the disease would permit the evaluation of the eustachian tube relatively free from these factors. In this section, findings of the eustachian tube studied in the convalescent stage of OME will be compared with those of the active stage to clarify primary and secondary factors of OME. Tests were performed with informed consent of patient's parent.

In the convalescent stage of OME, ventilatory and clearance functions of the tube were examined in 32 ears of children (4–9 years old). All of them showed no signs of the disease by inspection of the eardrum, audiometry, and tympanometry for 6 months after the treatment.

Fig. 5.6. Clearance function of tube in 230 ears with OME

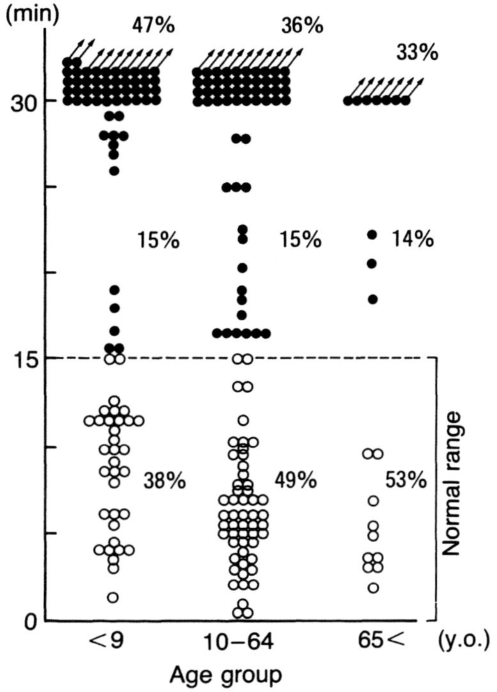

Second, mucosal changes of the middle ear in the convalescent stage were examined by endoscopy and were compared with those of the active stage to reveal the inflammatory factor in this disease. Endoscopy of the middle ear through the perforated eardrum was performed in 13 ears using a needle endoscope with a diameter of 1.7 mm (Selfoscope SES 1711K, Olympus, Tokyo, Japan). The images of the middle ear were recorded on a videotape through a TV camera (CCD camera DXC-1011, Sony, Tokyo, Japan) and compared with those of 26 ears in the active stage.

5.2.1 Is Eustachian Tube Function Impaired in Convalescent Stage of OME?

In the convalescent stage of OME, the opening pressure of the tube was found to be within the normal range in 91% of cases, which is 7% higher than in the active stage of the disease (Fig. 5.7). Stenosis of the tube noted in about 8% of cases in the active stage disappeared completely in the convalescent stage, probably owing to the decrease of mucosal edema or viscous fluid in the tube. These findings again indicate the absence of organic stenosis of the eustachian tube in the initial stage of OME.

Dynamic function of the tube to relieve positive pressure during swallowing was found to be improved markedly from 35.6% in the active stage to 50.0% in the convalescent stage (Fig. 5.8). This improvement is also considered to be due to the disappearance of inflammatory factors in the tube concomitantly with

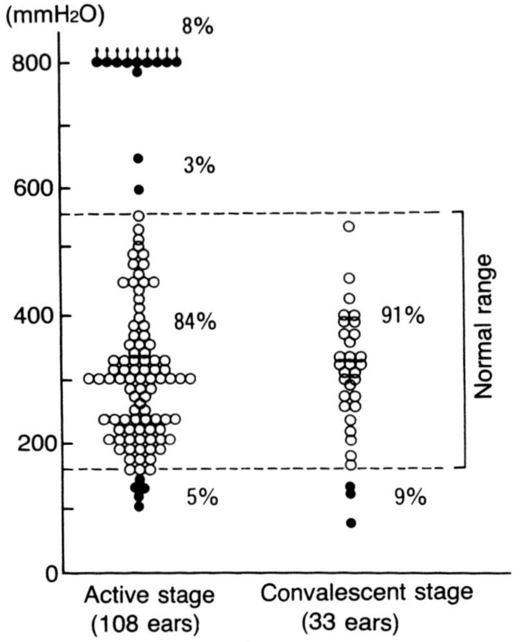

Fig. 5.7. Opening pressure of tube in active and convalescent stages of OME

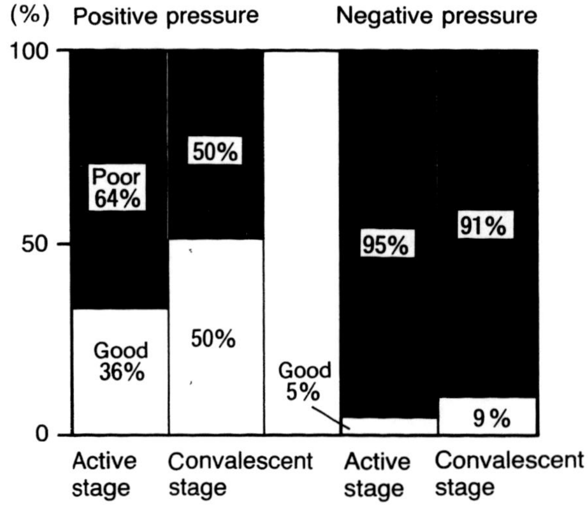

Fig. 5.8. Dynamic function of tube in active and convalescent stages of OME

improvement in the pathological condition of OME. In the negative pressure test, however, the tubal function in the convalescent stage was still impaired in 90.6% of cases, indicating little improvement of this function. Almost total loss of the tubal function in relieving negative pressure by swallowing, even in the convalescent stage, suggests that this impairment is a primary or predisposing factor of OME rather than a secondary one.

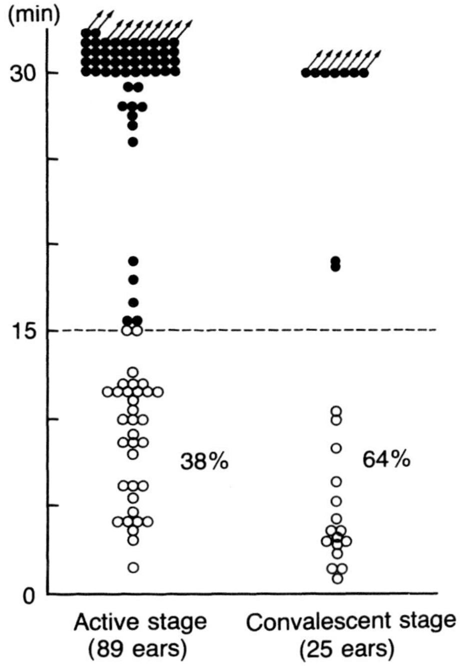

Fig. 5.9. Clearance function of tube in active and convalescent stages of OME

With respect to the clearance function of the tube, a marked improvement to 64.0% was observed in the convalescent stage (Fig. 5.9). Since the clearance function reflects the ciliary activity of the tube, the improvement appears to indicate disappearance of inflammation in the tubal mucosa.

When the eustachian tube functions were compared between the active and convalescent stages of OME (Fig. 5.10), the clearance function showed the greatest improvement (25.8%), followed by relief of positive pressure during swallowing (14.4%). Although improvement in opening pressure of the tube was only found in 8.3% of cases, this figure is of little significance since the result in the active stage was already normal in 84%. Relief of negative pressure in the convalescent stage, however, showed no appreciable improvement (4.6%) from the almost total loss of the function in the active stage. The inability of the tube to relieve any negative pressure showed no improvement even in the convalescent stage, indicating that this tubal dysfunction is not a secondary factor of OME but a predisposing one.

5.2.2 Is Tympanic Mucosa in Convalescent Stage Different from in Active Stage?

Endoscopic examination of the middle ear in the convalescent stage revealed no signs of inflammation such as edema or hyperemia of the mucosa, though mucosal vessels generally remained dilated (Figs. 5.11, 5.12). By contrast, in the active stage, edema (73.1%) or hyperemia (23.1%) of the mucosa were noted in nearly all patients, and the tympanic orifice of the tube was narrowed by surrounding

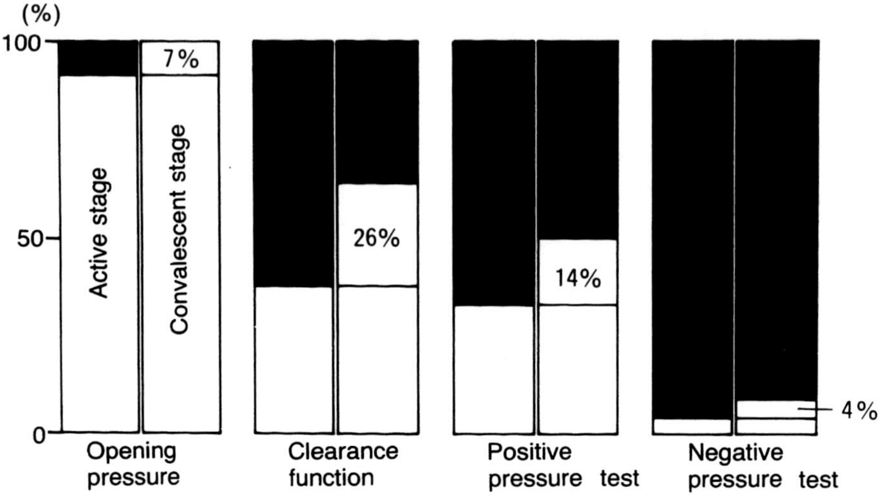

Fig. 5.10. Improvement of tubal functions in convalescent stage compared with those in active stage of OME

marked edema or mucus. These endoscopic findings of the ear suggested a close relation between OME and inflammation.

High prostaglandin levels in the middle ear effusion of OME patients have been reported by Bernstein et al. (1976) and Dennis et al. (1976). Prostaglandin E_2 levels in adults (18 ears) and children (23 ears) with OME were compared in this study to determine the degree of inflammation in OME in each age-group. In children, the prostaglandin E_2 level was significantly higher than in adults (Fig. 5.13), indicating the involvement of inflammation in the development of OME in children. However, the prostaglandin level in adult patients was 5 to over 100 times higher than the normal plasma level, which indicates that the inflammatory factor cannot be excluded in the development of adult OME.

Since inflammatory changes in the middle ear mucosa, such as edema and hyperemia including the tubal orifice, completely disappeared in the convalescent stage of OME, the eustachian tube is considered to be initially patent without any stenosis. This observation was consistent with the test results of tubal function in the previous section.

5.2.3 Cause of OME with Respect to Eustachian Tube in Convalescent Stage

In light of the above findings, the condition of the one-way valve or inability of the tube to relieve negative middle ear pressure appears to be a causative factor in the development of OME. As the middle ear pressure in OME is generally negative, this characteristic feature of tubal dysfunction has great significance in a closed ear space. However, no fluid retention was observed in the convalescent stage of OME, indicating that dysfunction of the eustachian tube is not the only factor responsible for development of OME. Thus, disorders of the tube appear to be necessary for the development of OME, though they are not sufficient in

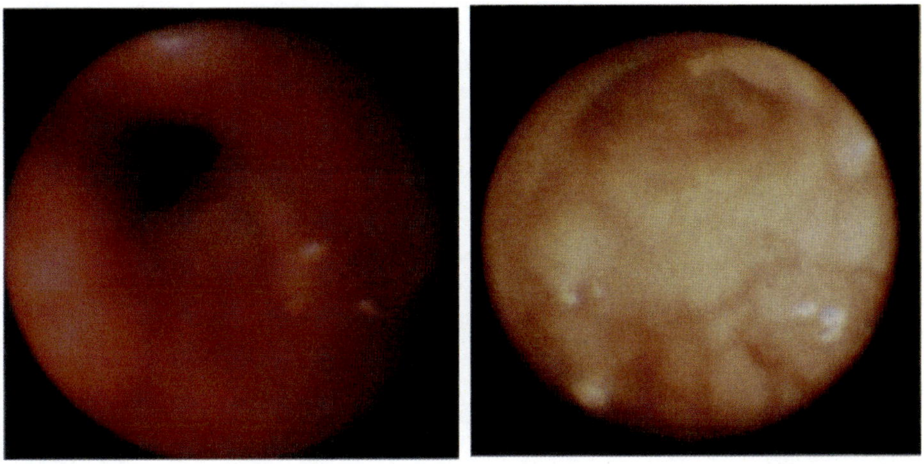

a b

Fig. 5.11a, b. Needlescopic findings of middle ear mucosa in OME. **a** Active stage with marked edema and hyperemia. **b** In convalescent stage, no sign of inflammation was noted

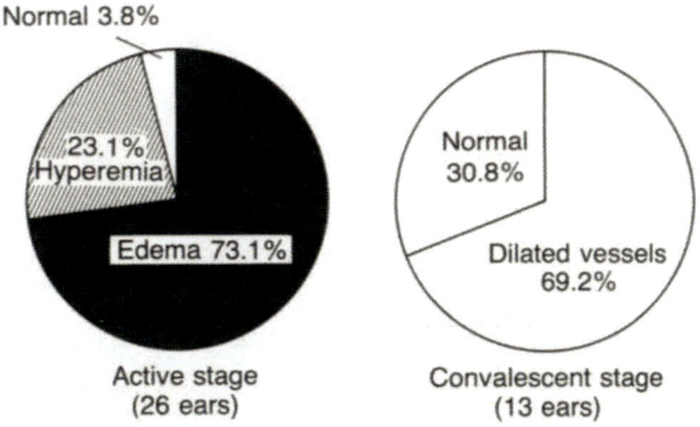

Fig. 5.12. Needlescopic findings of middle ear mucosa in OME

themselves. Involvement of other factors, such as the production of effusion or reduction in the middle ear pressure, is necessary for the development of the disease. These factors will be discussed in the following sections.

5.2.4 Summary

Eustachian tube functions and endoscopic findings of middle ear mucosa in the convalescent stage of OME (55 ears) were compared with those in the active stage (134 ears). The results were as follows:

a) The clearance function of the eustachian tube was markedly improved in the convalescent stage, followed by the relief of positive pressure during swallowing. The opening pressure of the tube in the convalescent stage indicated

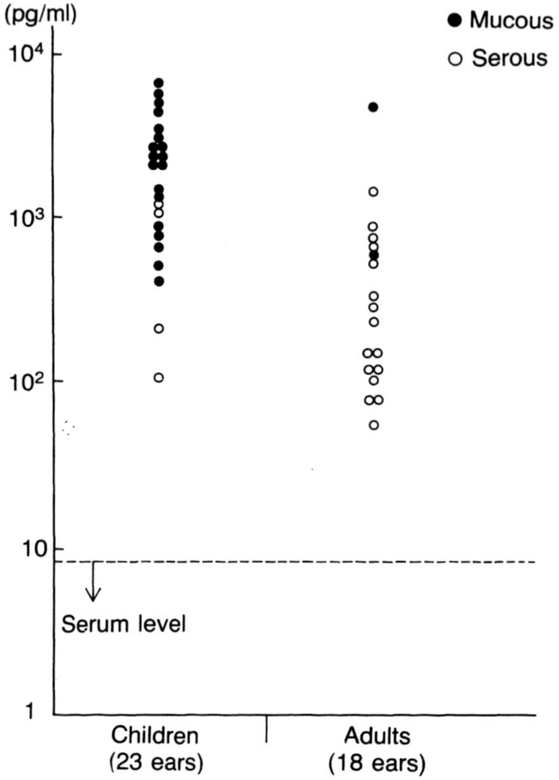

Fig. 5.13. Prostaglandin E_2 in middle ear effusion

complete disappearance of the tubal stenosis. Thus, tubal obstruction, which had been regarded as a cause of OME, was found to be a result of the disease.

b) The results of the negative pressure test, on the other hand, remained unchanged in most of the patients even in the convalescent stage. This impairment was, therefore, considered to be a primary and irreversible factor in OME.

c) Endoscopy of the tympanic cavity showed the complete disappearance of edema or hyperemia of the mucosa in the convalescent stage, indicating the involvement of inflammation in the development of OME.

5.3 Middle Ear Pressure in OME

The present study revealed that the eustachian tube in OME is unable to relieve negative middle ear pressure. At the same time, the middle ear pressure in OME has been regarded as being negative due to the retracted eardrum (Fig. 5.14) or from the C-type tympanogram at its early or convalescent stage. However, in the active stage of OME, determination of the middle ear pressure is rather difficult, because the ear generally shows a B-type tympanogram. In the present study,

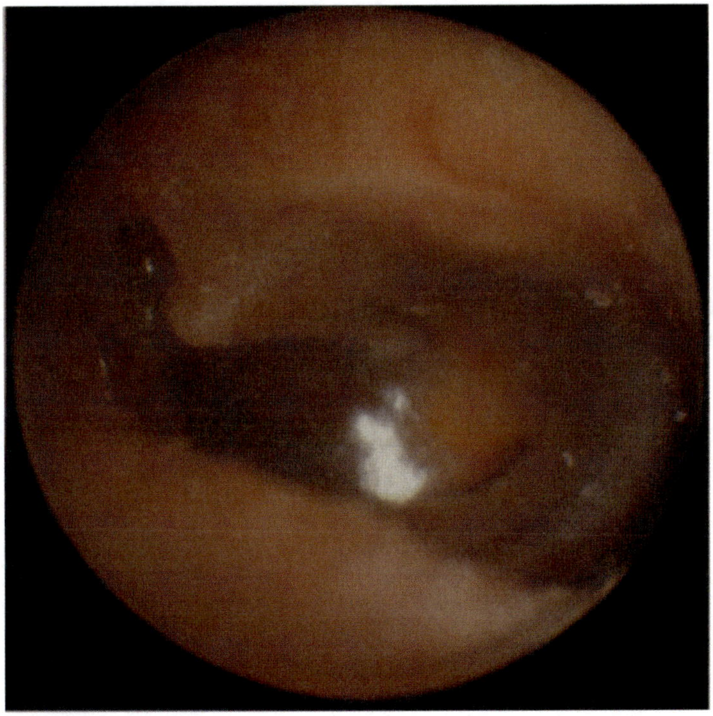

Fig. 5.14. Retracted eardrum in OME

direct measurement of the middle ear pressure was attempted before myringotomy for placement of tympanostomy tube in children.

The measurement was performed in 30 ears under general anesthesia with less than 30% O_2 and without N_2 to minimize gas production in the closed ear space. A fine flexible pressure transducer (Mikro-tip PC-330 3F, Miller Instr. Inc, Texas, USA) with a diameter of 1 mm (Fig. 5.15) was used. A pressure sensor at the tip of the transducer was advanced into the middle ear through the pharyngeal orifice of the tube via a ventilation catheter (Fig. 5.16). There was slight resistance when the transducer passed the tubal isthmus, and the entry of the sensor into the ear space could be confirmed by a synchronous increase in the pressure with compression of the eardrum from outside (Fig. 5.17).

The middle ear pressure in OME patients was found to range from +40 to −185 mmH_2O (Fig. 5.18). It was negative in 76.7% (23 ears) and positive in 16.7% (five ears). The mean value of the middle ear pressure was slightly negative (−54.0 mmH_2O). These results are in close agreement with those of transtympanic measurement of middle ear pressure (Kawabata et al. 1985). Thus, it was confirmed that the tympanic pressure was generally negative even in the presence of effusion in the middle ear.

This negative pressure appears puzzling because one would expect the middle ear to be positive when filled with fluid. The negative middle ear pressure had

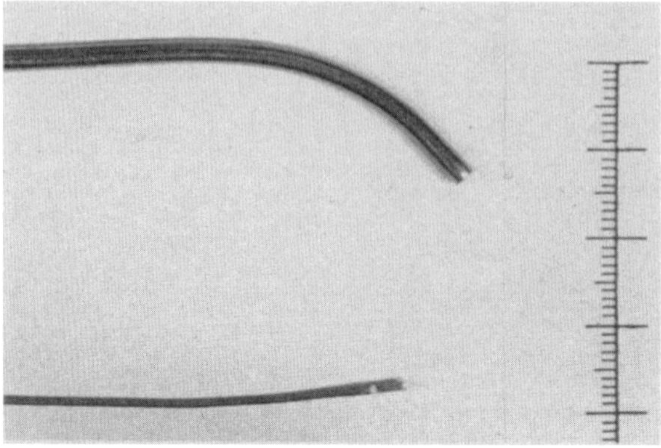

Fig. 5.15. Ventilation catheter (*above*) and fine flexible pressure transducer (*below*) for measurement of middle ear pressure

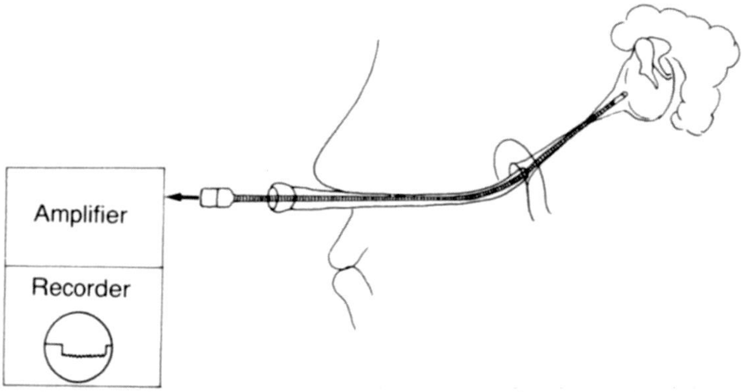

Fig. 5.16. Method for measuring middle ear pressure through eustachian tube

been considered to be a result of gas absorption by obliteration of the eustachian tube. However, as the present study excluded stenosis of the tube, the process producing negative middle ear pressure must be sought elsewhere. The presence of the negative pressure in the middle ear appears to be one of the etiological factors in the development of OME. The process by which negative middle ear pressure develops and the validity of the "hydrops ex vacuo" theory will be discussed in the following secton.

5.3.1 Summary

The middle ear pressure was measured directly through the eustachian tube in 30 ears with OME. In general, the middle ear was under slight negative pressure of less than -100 mmH_2O, even when fluid was retained. Negative middle ear pressure may contribute to the development of OME.

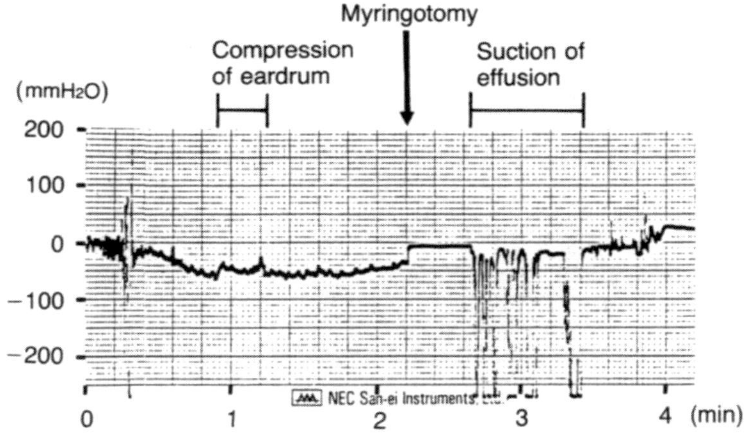

Fig. 5.17. Middle ear pressure in a 6-year-old boy with OME

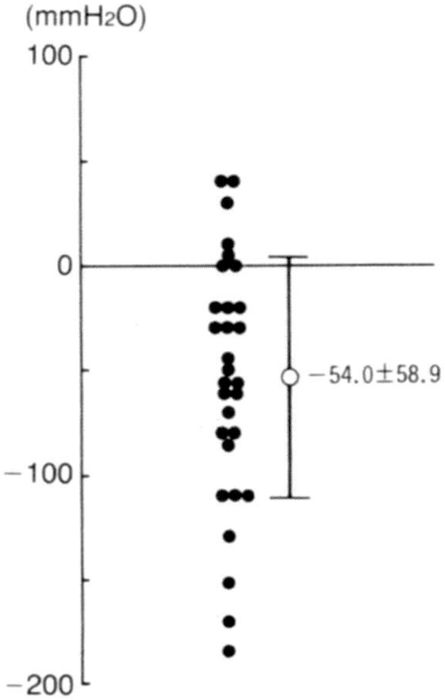

Fig. 5.18. Middle ear pressure in OME (30 ears)

5.4 "Hydrops Ex Vacuo" Theory in OME

The validity of the hydrops ex vacuo theory in the development of OME is examined in this section using experimental and clinical methods. According to this theory, the negative pressure develops in the middle ear due to absorption of gas when the middle ear becomes a closed cavity by obstruction of the tube. Effusion is then produced in the middle ear to compensate for the negative pressure. This theory has been supported by experimental findings whereby serous or bloody effusion was produced in the middle ear by sudden and high

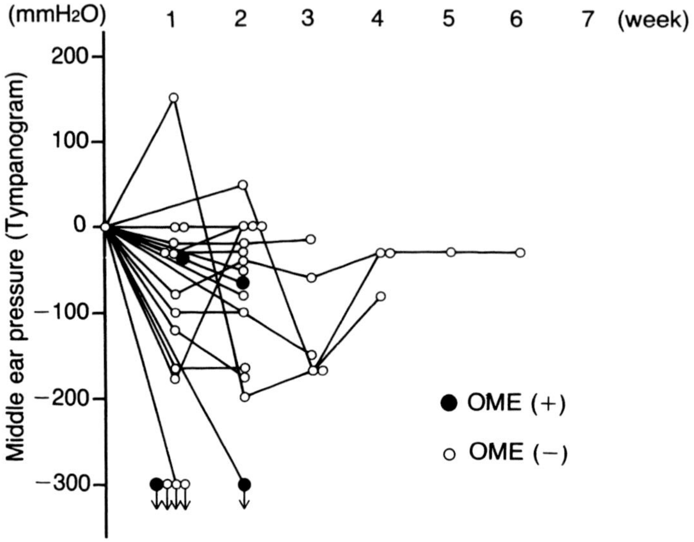

Fig. 5.19. Middle ear pressure after suppression of tubal ventilatory function in cats

negative pressure in the ear, as well as by the clinical experience of effusion in the ear caused by a marked pressure change in aerotitis media. However, the present studies revealed the absence of organic obstruction of the eustachian tube in OME. Therefore, as the next step, the validity of the hydrops ex vacuo theory was examined.

5.4.1 Experimentally Impaired Dynamic Function of Eustachian Tube

Functional obstruction of the tube was produced in cats (20 ears) by both cutting the tensor muscle and removing the hamulus pterygoideus, or destroying the trigeminal motor nuclei, with minimum invasion to the middle ear and eustachian tube. These procedures resulted in a negative pressure of less than −200 mmH_2O in the middle ear in many of the animals (Fig. 5.19), but retention of effusion was observed only in 3 of the 20 ears, suggesting that fluid retention is rarely caused by functional obstruction of the tube (Fig. 5.20). From these findings, hydrops ex vacuo by impairment of ventilatory function of the tube is unlikely, though this type of tubal disturbance is frequent in OME patients.

5.4.2 Experimental Formation of "Hydrops Ex Vacuo"

Next, negative middle ear pressure required for the production of effusion was examined experimentally in five cats. No effusion was observed at a middle ear pressure of −200 mmH_2O. The production of effusion was first noted when a pressure of −300 mmH_2O was applied to the ear for 4 h or more (Fig. 5.21). The hydrops ex vacuo theory appears to be valid only when high negative pressures for a certain period are applied to the closed ear space.

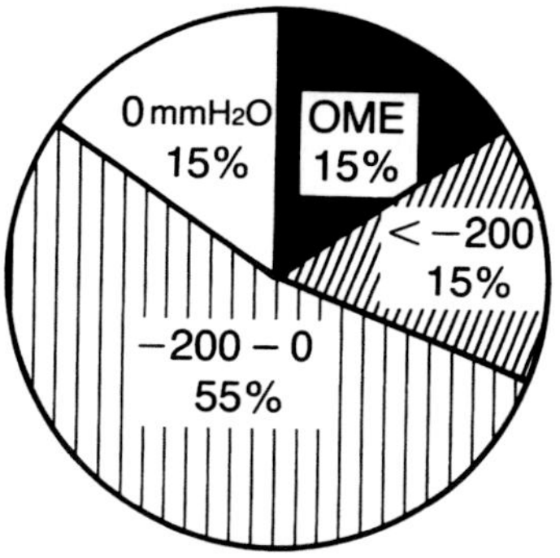

Fig. 5.20. Results of abolishing tubal ventilatory function in cats

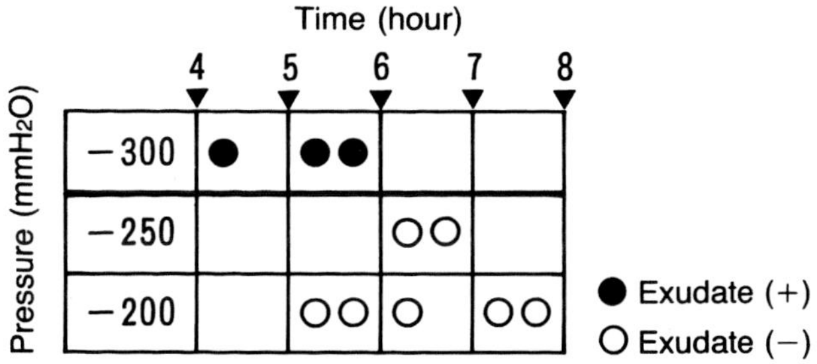

Fig. 5.21. Middle ear exudation induced by high negative pressure in cats

5.4.3 Sniff-Induced OME

With regard to the process of inducing high negative pressure in the ear under normal conditions, the only conceivable way is by sniffing. Negative middle ear pressure by sniffing would develop through the eustachian tube with closing failure when the tube is closed immediately after sniffing. The frequency of such a condition was examined in children with OME.

Of 100 children with OME who were asked whether they sniffed often or not, 66 replied that they did. Among them, 40 children were examined through the perforated eardrum to determine whether negative pressure was induced in the middle ear by sniffing. It was found that 12 of the children (14 ears) developed negative pressure by sniffing (Fig. 5.22). Although this negative pressure was two to five times greater when there was no tympanic perforation, closing of the tube after sniffing was observed only in ten children (12 ears). Therefore, development of negative pressure in the ear by sniffing was observed in only 17% of the OME patients examined. Thus, this process was not regarded as playing a primary role in the development of OME.

5.4.4 Summary

The validity of the hydrops ex vacuo theory in OME was evaluated experimentally and clinically, and it was excluded as the primary factor in the pathogenesis of OME.

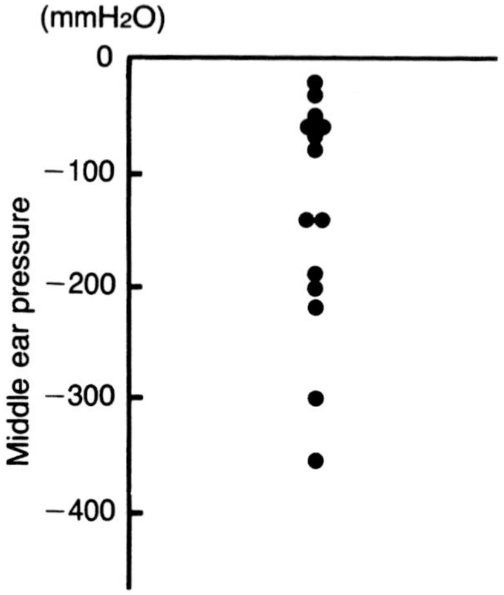

Fig. 5.22. Negative middle ear pressure induced by sniffing in children with OME

a) Functional disorders of the eustachian tube do not produce middle ear effusion, even in the presence of negative middle ear pressure.
b) Effusion was not produced unless a middle ear pressure of −300 mmH_2O was maintained for more than 4 h.
c) Sniff-induced negative middle ear pressure was infrequent and may not be the main cause of OME.

5.5 Development of Negative Middle Ear Pressure by Clearance of Eustachian Tube

The present results have shown that negative middle ear pressure and prolonged retention of fluid in OME patients cannot be explained by the hydrops ex vacuo theory. Murphy (1979) reported that mucus introduced into the closed ear of the cat produced a negative pressure due to ciliary clearance of the tube. Nozoe et al. (1984) found that muscular clearance, which was inhibited by negative pressure, recovered with the removal of the negative pressure. In reference to these studies, the formation of negative middle ear pressure by the clearance function of the tube was examined in cats by filling the ear with fluid to simulate OME.

5.5.1 Is Middle Ear Pressure Reduced by Ciliary Clearance?

Reduction in the middle ear pressure by ciliary clearance was examined in 12 cats (16 ears). The animals were anesthetized with ketamine hydrochloride and sodium pentobarbital under controlled respiration. A small hole made in the tympanic bulla was tightly connected to a polyvinyl tube. The middle ear was filled with saline solution, and the other end of the polyvinyl tube was connected to a micropressure transducer (Microtip PC-330 3F, Miller Instruments Inc, Texas, USA; Fig. 5.23a).

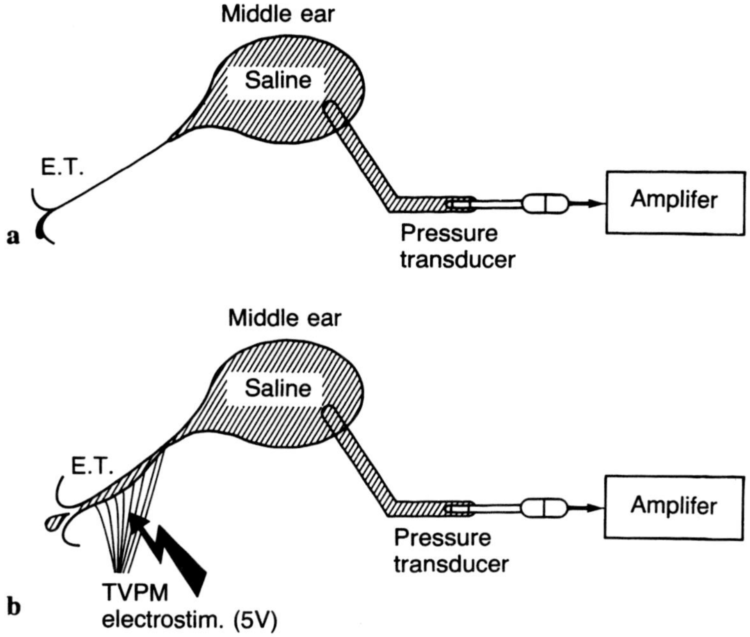

Fig. 5.23a, b. Development of negative middle ear pressure by tubal clearance function. **a** Ciliary clearance; **b** muscular clearance. *TVPM* tensor veli palatini muscle, *ET* eustachian tube

It was found that a pressure of -25 to -265 mmH_2O (mean -150.7 mmH_2O) was produced in all cases within 1–6 h, as shown in Fig. 5.24. In the most rapid case, a pressure of -170 mmH_2O was noted after 1 h, and a maximum negative pressure of -265 mmH_2O was produced about 3 h after instillation of the fluid in the ear. Such marked negative pressure, however, was slightly reduced after a few hours, probably by fluid secretion from the mucosa due to the high negative pressure in the ear. Consequently, the final middle ear pressure was around -150 mmH_2O, despite fluid retention in the middle ear space.

5.5.2 Is Middle Ear Pressure Reduced by Muscular Clearance?

Negative pressure produced by muscular activity of the tube was measured in seven cats (nine ears) in the same way as in the above experiment. To simulate swallowing, contraction of the tensor muscle was induced by electric stimulation (5 V) at intervals of 10–15 s and the middle ear pressure was recorded (Fig. 5.23b). The pressure was reduced at each tensor contraction in a steplike pattern, as shown in Fig. 5.25. In this animal, a pressure of -55 mmH_2O developed in the ear in about 3 min. The pressure reduction due to muscular activity reached a maximum level of -10 to -60 mmH_2O after 10–20 contractions of the tensor in the presence of fluid in the middle ear.

The mean maximum negative pressures by ciliary and muscular clearance

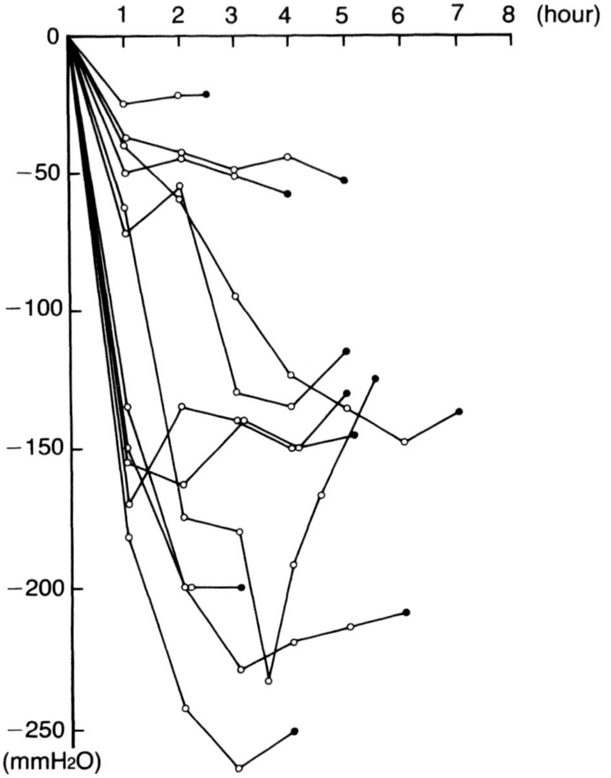

Fig. 5.24. Negative middle ear pressure induced by ciliary clearance in 16 cat ears

were −150.7 mmH_2O (at 3.3 h) and −27.0 mmH_2O (at 3 min; Fig. 5.26). These studies revealed that a marked negative pressure is produced by ciliary activity within a few hours, while a slight negative pressure results from muscular activity in a few minutes.

5.5.3 Development of Negative Middle Ear Pressure in OME

When fluid is present in the closed middle ear cavity, the clearance of the fluid from the tube decreases the middle ear pressure. These characteristic findings may provide an important key in clarifying the pathogenesis of OME. Fluid filling the middle ear and mastoid cavity in OME patients is clearly demonstrated by magnetic resonance imaging (MRI; Fig. 5.27). Such a condition leads to the development of negative middle ear pressure by the clearance function of the tube. However, negative pressure is not observed in the ear with acute suppurative otitis media, presumably because of the impaired clearance of the tube by inflammation and the rapid production of effusion. Slow production of effusion with intact ciliary activity is a necessary condition for the reduction in middle ear pressure. In patients with OME, however, the negative middle

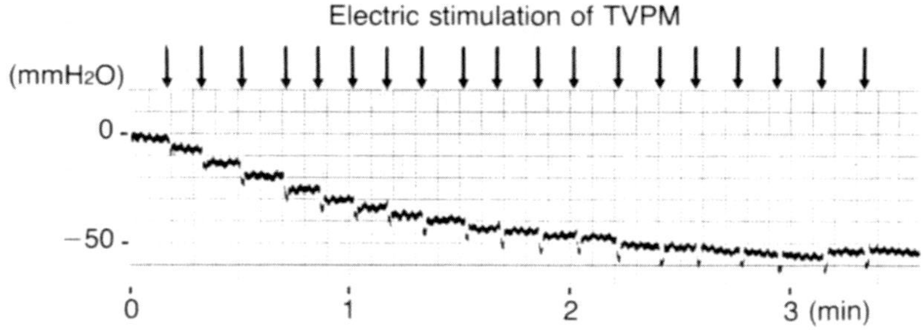

Fig. 5.25. Negative middle ear pressure induced by muscular clearance in cats

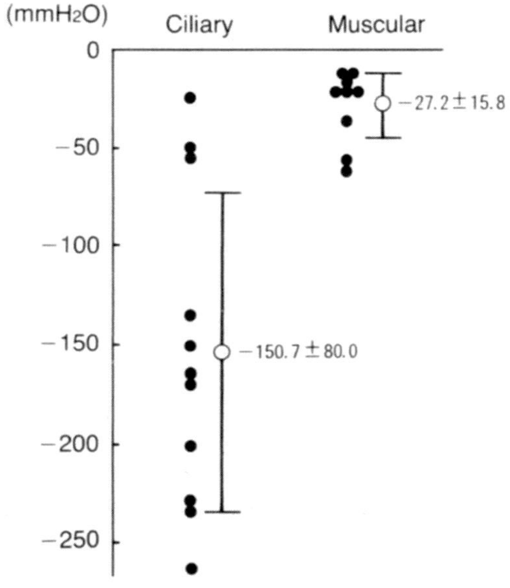

Fig. 5.26. Maximum negative middle ear pressure due to tubal clearance function

ear pressure cannot be relieved by swallowing due to the impaired dynamic function of the tube. Thus, an irreversible condition of negative pressure concurrent with fluid retention develops in the closed cavity.

5.5.4 Summary

The extent of reduction in the middle ear pressure due to ciliary and muscular clearance of the tube was examined in 19 cats after filling the middle ear with saline solution. The results were as follows:

a) A maximum pressure of −25 to −265 mmH_2O (mean −150.7 mmH_2O) developed in the middle ear by the ciliary activity within 1–6 h (mean 3.3 h).
b) A negative middle ear pressure of −10 to −60 mmH_2O (mean −27.2 mmH_2O) was produced by the muscular activity in a few minutes after simulated swallowing of 10–20 times.

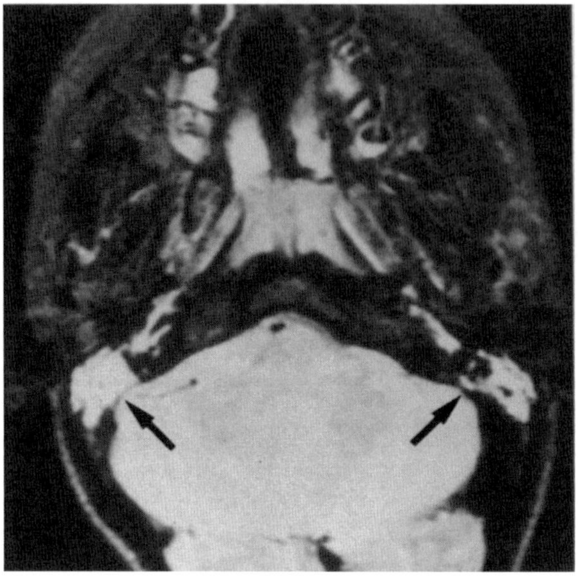

Fig. 5.27. MRI of an 11-year-old child with bilateral OME. Middle ear cavities of both sides are filled with effusion (*arrows*)

5.6 Ventilation of Middle Ear and Clearance of Eustachian Tube

The present studies revealed that the middle ear pressure in OME becomes negative by ciliary and muscular activity of the tube when the eardrum is intact. In addition, clinical studies demonstrated that the eustachian tube of OME patients cannot relieve this negative pressure by swallowing. Based on these characteristic findings, a study was made as to whether clearance of fluid is delayed when the ventilatory function of the tube is experimentally impaired.

In 13 ears of seven cats, the middle ear was filled with saline solution and closed tightly. The ventilatory function of the tube was suppressed in seven ears by both cutting the tensor muscle and removing the hamulus pterygoideus, while the remaining six ears were left intact as normal controls. After 2–7 days, the amount of fluid remaining in the middle ear was examined (Fig. 5.28). In all of the control ears, the fluid was expelled, while in six of seven ears with tubal dysfunction 0.1–0.5 cm^3 fluid remained. Middle ear pressure in one of the ears with tubal damage was -150 mmH_2O, which was compatible with the negative pressure developed by the ciliary clearance in the former experiment. These findings strongly suggest that when fluid is retained in the middle ear with poor ventilatory function of the tube, transtubal clearance of the fluid is markedly delayed by irreversible negative pressure in the middle ear.

If OME is improved by ventilating the middle ear through the perforated eardrum, the closed condition of the middle ear cavity will be a pathogenetic factor in OME. This possibility was examined clinically.

The negative middle ear pressure in 53 ears of 40 patients with OME (age

Fig. 5.28. Amount of middle ear fluid remaining after destruction of tubal ventilatory function

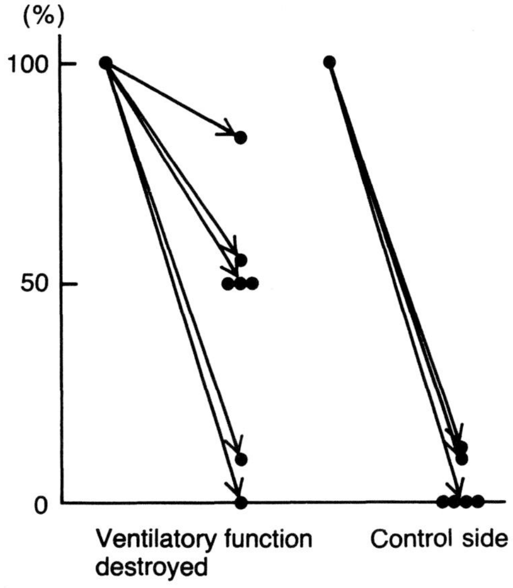

3–53 years) was relieved by myringotomy without aspirating the fluid. The fluid was observed under a microscope. Examinations were made 1 h or 1 day after myringotomy, and the property of the effusion was examined at the same time. In patients examined 1 h after the operation, the eustachian tube function was examined in the manner described in the previous section.

5.6.1 One Hour After Myringotomy

In 10 of 30 ears examined, the fluid had disappeared 1 h after myringotomy (Fig. 5.29) regardless of whether the effusion was serous or mucous. Of the 13 ears, 12 showed normal opening pressure, suggesting the absence of any stenosis of the tube, but none of the ears were capable of reducing negative middle ear pressure by swallowing. The clearance time was within 15 min (normal) in some ears but delayed in others, showing no definite correlation between the disappearance of fluid and the clearance function of the eustachian tube.

5.6.2 One Day After Myringotomy

In 24 of 30 ears, the fluid had disappeared 1 day after the myringotomy, but the relation between this finding and the property of the fluid was also obscure.

The drainage of middle ear fluid in the early stage after myringotomy is considered to depend mainly on muscular activity and to a lesser extent on ciliary activity. The immediate relief of the negative middle ear pressure by myringotomy is considered to restore the clearance function of the eustachian tube at an early stage. These clinical findings indicate that drainage of the fluid is delayed by reduction of the ear pressure following clearance of the tube. However, when the negative pressure was normalized by myringotomy, transtubal drainage of the fluid was restored immediately.

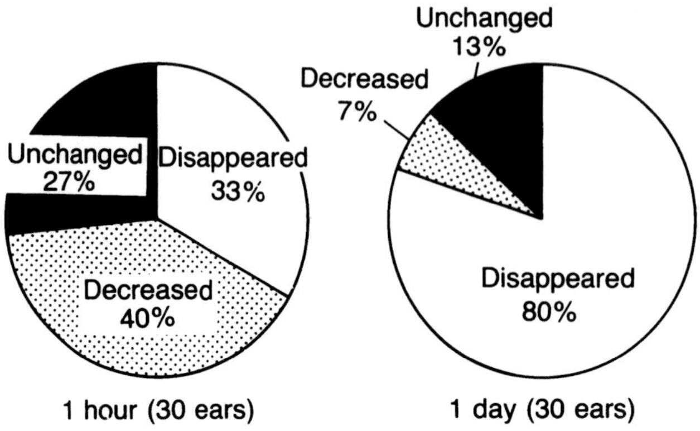

Fig. 5.29. Middle ear effusion after myringotomy

5.6.3 Summary

Myringotomy was performed in 53 ears of children with OME to observe the extent of drainage of the middle ear fluid. The fluid had disappeared in 33% of cases 1 h after the procedure and in 80% after 1 day. These findings strongly suggest that the clearance function of the tube was promptly restored by the normalization of middle ear pressure by myringotomy, allowing drainage of the fluid out of the ear.

5.7 Experimental OME

The former experiments revealed that if fluid is retained in the middle ear with an impaired eustachian tube function, drainage of the fluid is delayed by reduction of the middle ear pressure. On the other hand, the condition of OME was found not to result from tubal dysfunction alone, but edematous middle ear mucosa and the high level of prostaglandin E_2 in the effusion suggested that inflammation producing middle ear effusion is the primary pathogenetic factor in the development of OME, especially in children.

There have been reports (DeMaria et al. 1984; Takasaka et al. 1984) on the production of experimental OME by introducing inflammatory agents into the middle ear, but the disease did not persist for a long period like actual OME. Therefore, the effect of inflammatory agents in the middle ear was evaluated together with impairment of the ventilatory function of the tube.

By cutting the tensor muscle and removing the hamulus pterygoideus, the dynamic function of the eustachian tube was suppressed in eight ears of eight cats. After 1–2 weeks, effusion in the middle ear was noted in only one ear. In the remaining seven ears, which did not develop OME despite functional obstruction of the tube, endotoxin of *Esherichia coli* (40–50 ng) was introduced into the ear once, or twice after a 1-week interval. Retention of effusion was observed in six ears (Fig. 5.30), and the condition persisted for a mean period of 6.3 weeks. Tympanographic changes in one of these ears are presented in Fig.

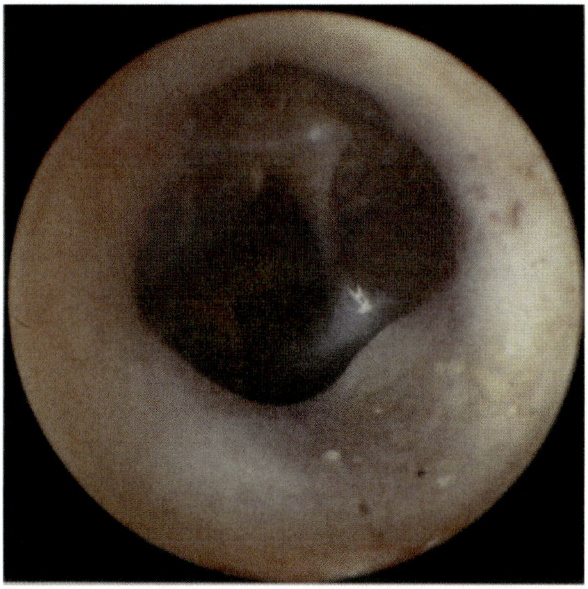

Fig. 5.30. Experimental OME in a cat

5.31, which shows a prolonged B-type tympanogram for 8 weeks after instilling the endotoxin. By contrast, in four ears in which the endotoxin was given two to four times without impairing the tubal function, effusion was observed in two ears, but it lasted only for a mean period of 1.5 weeks (Fig. 5.32).

This experiment indicates that OME develops and is prolonged by a combination of impairment of the tubal function and fluid production in the ear. Loss of dynamic function of the eustachian tube and the inflammatory process in the middle ear are considered to constitute essential pathological conditions in persistent OME.

5.8 Pathogenesis of OME

The pathological process of OME with respect to the eustachian tube may be summarized as follows. Since stenosis or obstruction of the eustachian tube is infrequent in patients with OME, hydrops ex vacuo is unlikely as an explanation of the pathogenesis of OME. However, the dynamic function of the eustachian tube to relieve negative pressure by swallowing was found to be lost in patients with OME. Since this type of tubal dysfunction persists in almost all patients in the convalescent stage of OME, it is considered to be a predisposing factor leading to the development of OME.

The middle ear pressure in OME patients is generally negative even when the middle ear is filled with fluid, and relief of this negative pressure by myringotomy results in early drainage of the fluid. Negative pressure in the closed middle ear cavity, therefore, appears to promote the development of OME. This negative middle ear pressure was found to be caused by the clearance of the fluid

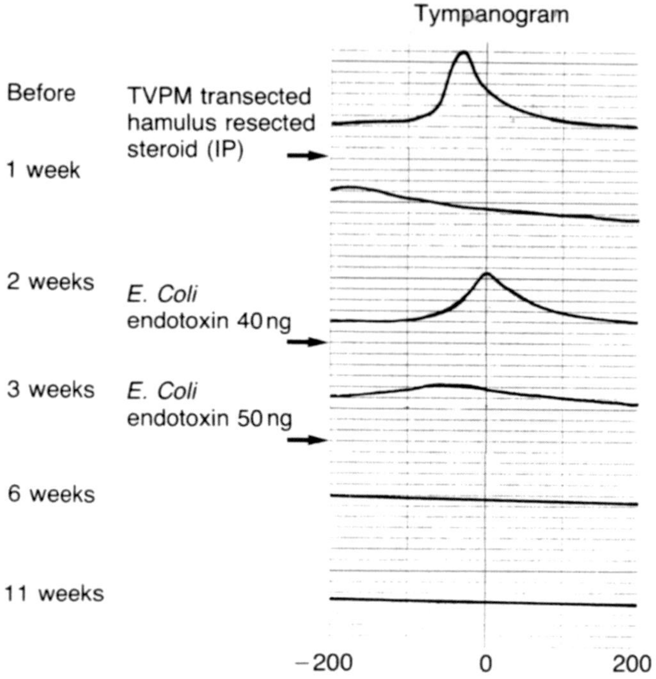

Fig. 5.31. Progression of experimental OME in a cat evaluated by tympanograms

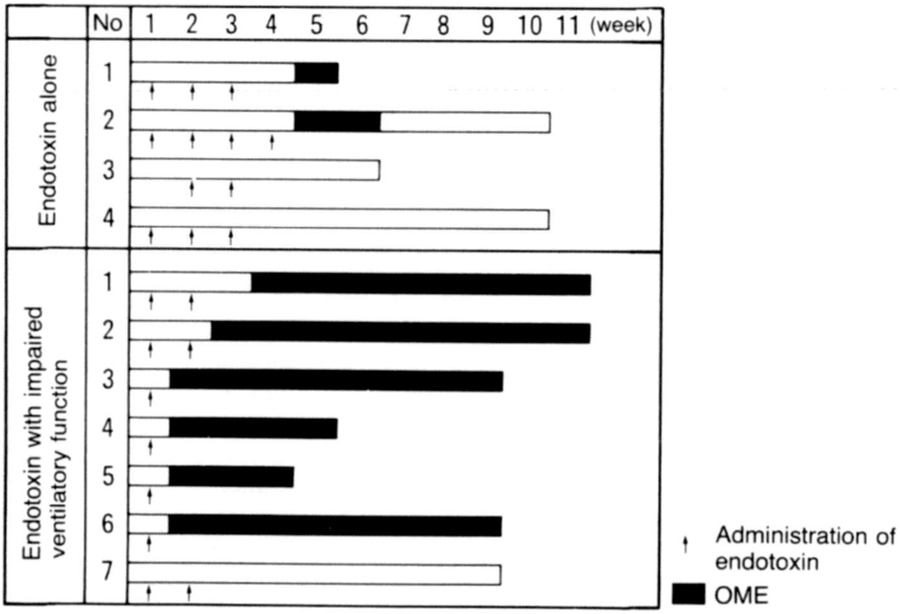

Fig. 5.32. Differences in course of experimental OME by either endotoxin alone or endotoxin with tubal disturbance

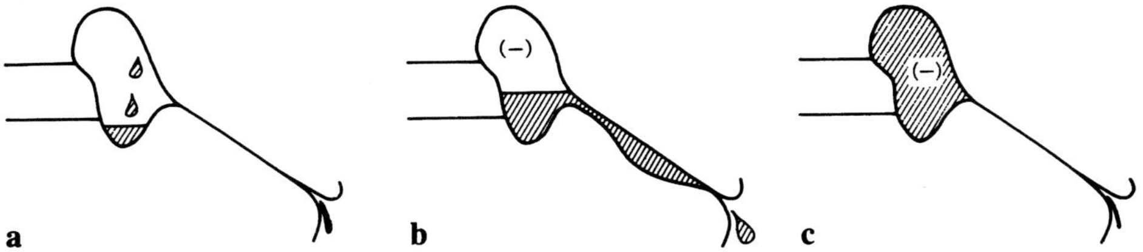

Fig. 5.33a–c. Development of OME. **a** Production of effusion and its ciliary clearance; **b** accumulation of effusion and its muscular clearance; **c** arrest of muscular clearance and diminishing of ciliary clearance, leading to development of OME

in the closed middle ear cavity.

These clinical and experimental observations suggest the following process in the development of OME. The eustachian tube of OME patients is defective as it is a one-way valve incapable of relieving negative pressure in the closed ear cavity. First, inflammation may cause production of fluid in the early stage of OME. Endoscopic observation of the middle ear mucosa and the prostaglandin E_2 level in the effusion support this inflammatory process. When effusion occurs in the middle ear, the ciliary activity of the tube drains the fluid, leading to reduction of the middle ear pressure at the same time. When production of the fluid exceeds the capacity of ciliary clearance, muscular clearance of the tube starts to work. Though this muscular clearance efficiently drains the fluid, the pressure in the closed middle ear cavity become rapidly negative with every act of swallowing. As the eustachian tube here is incapable of relieving this negative pressure, the muscular activity ceases when the negative pressure exceeds a certain level. Ciliary activity of the tube, which is less affected by the negative pressure, is maintained to reduce the middle ear pressure (Fig. 5.33). However, this ciliary clearance finally diminishes, resulting in fluid remaining in the middle ear concurrently with negative pressure in the ear. Thus, the prolonged condition of OME, namely retention of fluid in the middle ear cavity under negative pressure, develops (Fig. 5.34).

5.9 Therapies for OME with Respect to Eustachian Tube

Considering the treatment of OME from the pathogenetic factors of the disease, a chain of events leading to the development of OME indicated above must be broken somewhere. As mentioned before, the primary pathological conditions of OME are both dysfunction of the eustachian tube and inflammation-induced effusion in the closed ear cavity. Impairment of the tubal function is regarded to be a predisposing factor that is difficult to correct. The treatment of OME, therefore, consists of reducing negative middle ear pressure and controlling the inflammation to minimize the effusion.

Since OME in children may be resolved spontaneously with age, radical or long-term treatment may not always be necessary. The emphasis in the treatment, therefore, should be placed on the improvement of hearing and preven-

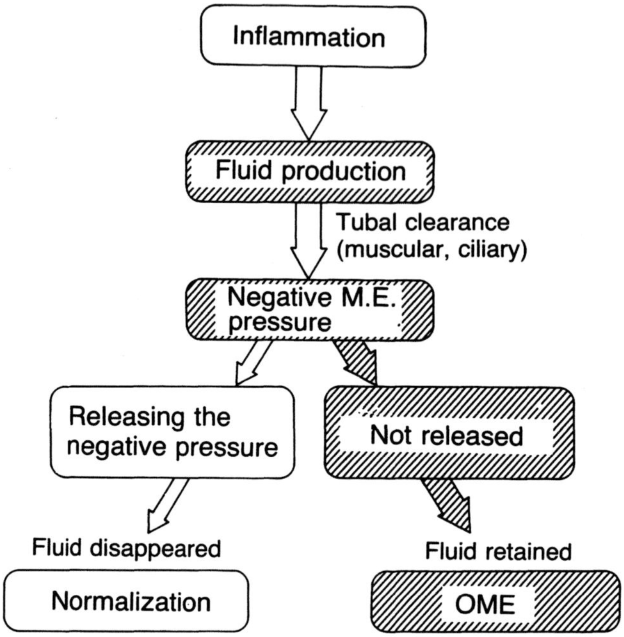

Fig. 5.34. Present concept of development of OME. *ME* Middle ear

tion of complications or sequelae. Various treatments of OME will be evaluated in relation to the eustachian tube in the following sections.

5.9.1 Effect of Inflation of Eustachian Tube

Inflation of the tube by a catheter or Politzer's maneuver is effective in relieving the negative middle ear pressure and promoting drainage of middle ear effusion through the tube. Inflation by catheter is a reliable procedure for inflating the tube. However, the normalization of middle ear pressure may be temporary, and the effect of the treatment appears to be limited. By MRI, the effectiveness of catheterization for drainage of effusion was examined in an 11-year-old boy. The amount of effusion judged by MRI was not different before and 1 week after three applications of the inflation therapy, suggesting that complete cure of OME is difficult using this procedure alone (Fig. 5.35).

Politzerization also has its shortcomings when evaluated in relation to the eustachian tube. About 78% of the children with OME were found to have rhinitis or nasal sinusitis, and endoscopy disclosed contamination or obstruction of the pharyngeal orifice of the tube by purulent nasal discharge in 72% of children with OME. Endoscopy of the nasopharynx revealed that this postnasal drip remains around the pharyngeal orifice of the tube even after aspiration through the nose. It may be pushed into the tube by inflation with Politzer's maneuver.

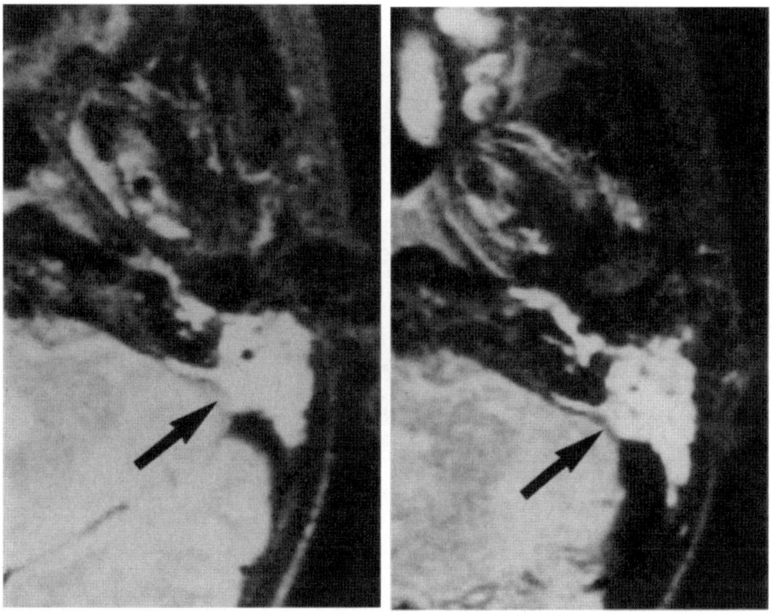

Fig. 5.35a, b. MRI middle ear effusion **a** before and **b** after air inflation. No change can be seen between the two (*arrows*)

5.9.1.1 Summary

Although inflation of the eustachian tube may be useful for temporary relief of negative middle ear pressure, it was found to have little effect on drainage of the middle ear effusion. Politzerization may be disadvantageous unless the nasal cavity is cleaned before the inflation.

5.9.2 Myringotomy and Insertion of Tympanostomy Tube in Eardrum

Perforation of the eardrum, either by myringotomy or insertion of the tube, effectively relieves the negative pressure in the ear with OME. These procedures achieve marked improvement in hearing and prompt drainage of middle ear effusion. However, the therapeutic effect of the two methods may be different because the duration of opening in the eardrum may differ markedly. The effects of the two methods in the treatment of OME were compared with respect to the recurrence rate of OME.

5.9.2.1 Recurrence of OME After Myringotomy

Myringotomy was performed in 35 ears and the recurrence of OME was examined 2, 4, and 6 months after surgery (Fig. 5.36). After 2 months, OME had recurred in 65.7% of ears. According to our observations, the perforation of the drum closes over a mean period of 10 days. Therefore, these eardrums were considered to have closed by the time of the first observation. The disease re-

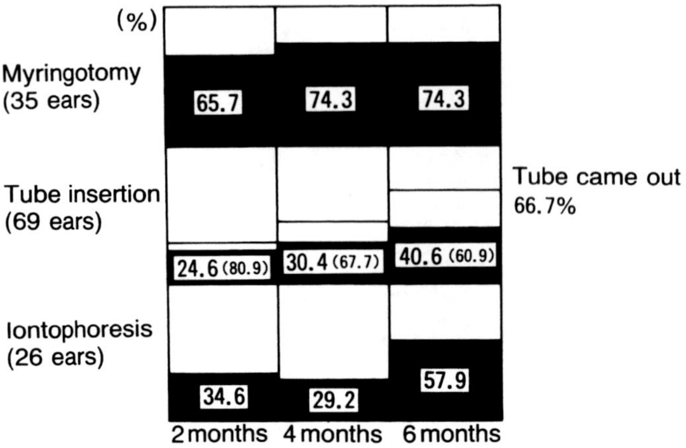

Fig. 5.36. Recurrence rates of OME after three different treatments. *Figures in parentheses* indicate recurrence rates in patients with tympanostomy tubes that came out

curred in 74.3% of ears after 4 and 6 months. The duration of the opening after myringotomy is considered to be insufficient for recovery from OME.

5.9.2.2 Recurrence of OME After Insertion of Tympanostomy Tube

The recurrence of OME was studied in 69 ears that underwent insertion of a tympanostomy tube as the initial treatment for OME. The recurrence rate was found to be markedly low in this group, being 24.6% after 2 months and 40.6% even after 6 months. No recurrence was observed when the tube remained in place. Among patients in whom the tube was displaced, however, OME recurred in 80.9% after 2 months, 67.7% after 4 months, and 60.9% after 6 months. In this group, recurrence was as high as in those patients who underwent myringotomy alone, indicating the importance of continuous ventilation of the ear through the perforation. OME appeared to be controlled in almost 60% of patients only by maintaining ventilation of the middle ear through a tympanostomy tube.

Since the recurrence rate decreased as the duration of insertion became longer, it appears advisable to keep the tube in place as long as possible. OME can be controlled as long as the tympanic cavity is ventilated through the hole in the eardrum. During this period, OME may be improved by restoration of both the clearance function of the tube and by normalization of the middle ear mucosa.

5.9.2.3 Summary

Although both myringotomy and a tympanostomy tube are effective for relief of the negative middle ear pressure in OME, this condition should be maintained for a certain period to resolve the disease. The recurrence rate of OME was 60%–70% in patients with myringotomy, which was maintained for only about 10 days. Insertion of a tympanostomy tube, on the other hand, showed a significantly lower rate of recurrence (40%) even 6 months after the procedure,

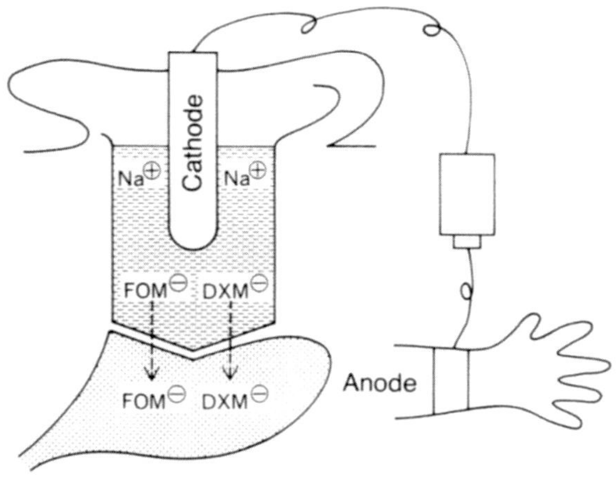

Fig. 5.37. Principle of iontophoresis treatment

including those patients in whom the tube had become displaced. Recurrence of OME was not observed as long as the tympanostomy tube remained in place.

5.9.3 Transtympanic Iontophoresis of Corticosteroids and Antibiotics

With respect to conservative therapy for OME, there are many reports on oral administration of corticosteroids or antibiotics. On the other hand, Passali et al. (1984) reported a method of treatment by transtympanic iontophoresis of carbocysteine. In reference to their report, the effectiveness of transtympanic iontophoresis of corticosteroids and antibiotics was examined experimentally and clinically (Fig. 5.37). The effectiveness of this treatment for OME patients was compared with that of oral administration of antibiotics.

5.9.3.1 Drug Passage Through Eardrum by Iontophoresis

As a preliminary study, the amount of drug transported from the external ear into the middle ear by iontophoresis was examined in 30 guinea pigs. A solution of corticosteroid (0.2% dexamethasone sodium phosphate) and an antibiotic (2% fosfomycin sodium) was instilled into the external ear canal, and iontophoresis was performed. The amount of the drugs transported through the eardrum was measured after 5, 10, and 15 min. The transport of dexamethasone was proportionate to the duration of the iontophoresis, and its concentration in the middle ear after 15 min of iontophoresis was 129.6 ± 45.2 ng.ml, which was sufficient for exhibiting an anti-inflammatory effect (Fig. 5.38).

The transport of fosfomycin was also proportionate to the time of iontophoresis, and its concentration in the middle ear was 38.9 ± 24.7 μg/ml (Fig. 5.39), which was sufficient to produce antimicrobial effects against *Hemophilus influenzae* and *Streptococcus pneumoniae*.

5.9.3.2 Effect of Iontophoresis in OME

In 13 children (22 ears, aged 3–6 years) with OME, a solution of 0.2% dexamethasone sodium phosphate and 2% fosfomycin sodium was ionto-

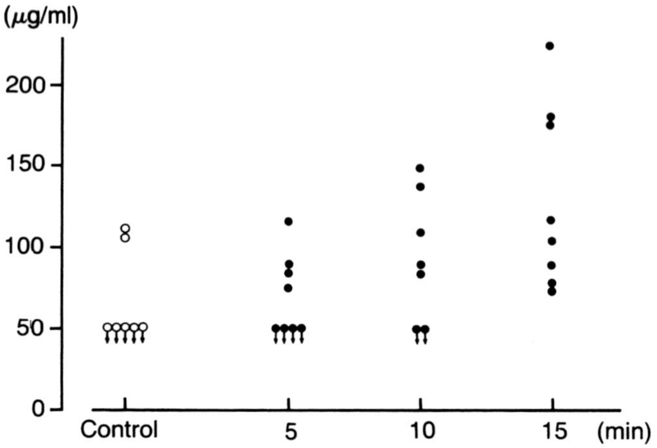

Fig. 5.38. Iontophoretic application of dexamethasone sodium phosphate into middle ear. Controls were given dexamethasone sodium phosphate for 15 min without iontophoresis. Reproduced from Sato et al (1988) Arch Otolaryngol 114:531–533. © 1988 American Medical Association

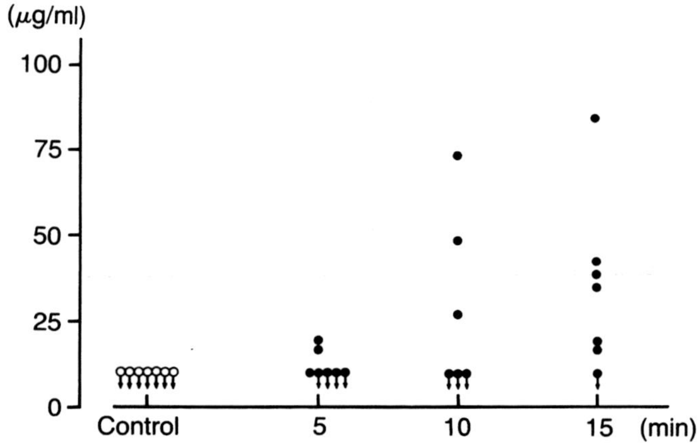

Fig. 5.39. Iontophoretic application of fosfomycin sodium into middle ear. Controls were given fosfomycin sodium for 15 min without iontophoresis. Reproduced from Sato et al (1988) Arch Otolaryngol 114:531–533. © 1988 American Medical Association

phoretically applied, ten times every 2 days for 15 min. Tympanometry and audiometry were performed before and 1 and 2 months after the treatment. The results were compared with children (27 ears, aged 3–7 years) with OME treated by oral administration of antibiotics (amoxicillin or cefaclor, 30–50 mg/kg for 2 weeks). As the control group, 17 untreated OME children (21 ears, aged 4–7 years) were examined.

The average hearing level at 500, 1000, and 2000 Hz is shown in Fig. 5.40. In the group treated by iontophoresis, the hearing improved markedly 1 month

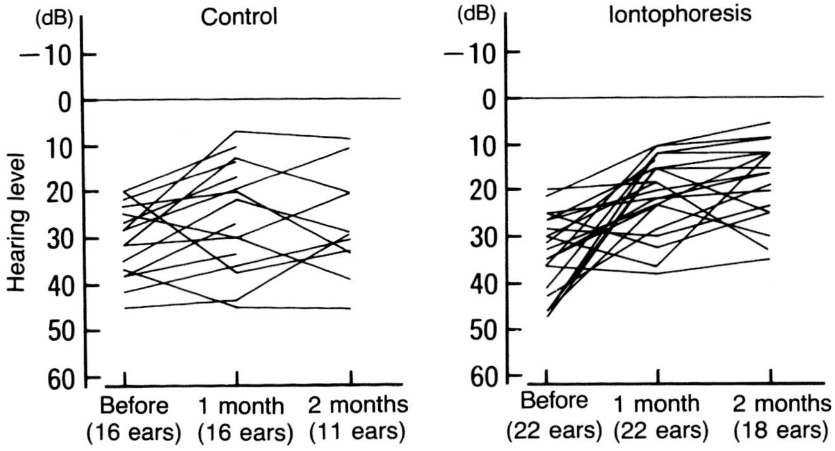

Fig. 5.40. Hearing improvement after iontophoresis treatment

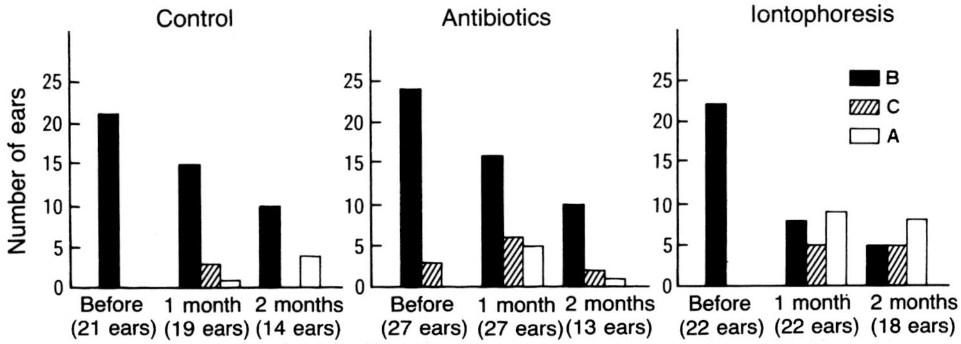

Fig. 5.41. Tympanogram findings with three different types of treatments

after the treatment and improved further after 2 months. Although hearing in the oral antibiotics group improved as compared with the control group 1 month after the treatment, the difference was not significant at 2 months. In the iontophoresis group, a significant improvement was noted after 2 months as compared with the control group, suggesting the long-standing effect of iontophoresis (Table 5.1).

Tympanograms were frequently of type B in the antibiotics group as in the control group both at 1 and 2 months, indicating little improvement of OME in these groups. However, the iontophoresis group 1 month after the treatment showed more type A than type B, suggesting a marked improvement in OME by this treatment with no deterioration of this condition at 2 months (Fig. 5.41).

As demonstrated in Sect 5.2.2, inflammation of the middle ear mucosa and high prostaglandin E_2 concentrations in the effusion indicate involvement of inflammation in the development of OME. Steroids and antibiotics transported to

Table 5.1. Difference of hearing improvement between treatments

	1 Month	2 Months
Control	5.32 ± 10.69^a	4.21 ± 11.88^a
Antibiotics	12.57 ± 6.66^a	8.57 ± 14.09
Iontophoresis	12.80 ± 12.96	16.76 ± 13.30^a

$^a p < 0.05$

the middle ear by this procedure appear to act on the middle ear mucosa to suppress production of effusion in the ear. The oral administration of these drugs was expected to suppress inflammation of the upper respiratory tract, including the nose and the eustachian tube, but the effects were found to be too short to allow recovery from OME.

5.9.3.3 Summary

a) Experimental studies revealed that iontophoresis of dexamethasone and fosfomycin transports drugs through the eardrum to the middle ear at concentrations sufficient for therapeutic effects.
b) Significant improvement of OME by iontophoresis was observed in OME children by audiometry and tympanometry, indicating the usefulness of this procedure for conservative treatment of young children with OME.

5.10 Summary of Chapter

It should be emphasized that patients with OME rarely have stenosis or obstruction of the eustachian tube. This characteristic finding requires major changes in the conventional concept related to the disease. However, the eustachian tube is still responsible for development of OME, since so-called functional obstruction of the tube, or locking by the negative middle ear pressure, was generally found in patients with OME.

When we consider the pathogenesis of this disease, it is of importance to understand how the three major characteristics of OME, namely fluid retention, negative middle ear pressure, and functional obstruction of the tube, are related to each other. The conventional concept of OME, whereby tubal obstruction initiates the formation of negative middle ear pressure, causing fluid retention, was found to be invalid with the finding that the tubal obstruction seldom occurs in OME patients. Also, negative pressure caused by sniffing was found to be infrequent.

Based on clinical and experimental data, the following process is considered to take place in the development of OME. The initial production of effusion causes negative middle ear pressure, which leads to functional obstruction of the eustachian tube. This process is the complete reverse of the conventional concept in explaining the pathogenesis of OME.

The middle ear cavity of OME patients resembles that of the embryo filled with amniotic fluid. The pathological condition of OME is, in a sense, a result of failure to maintain the middle ear in an aerated cavity, which is essential for an auditory organ in the air. Maintenance of the middle ear cavity in an aerated condition by the eustachian tube is difficult, especially in infants. The pathological condition of OME may represent a pitfall in the evolutionary process to acquire hearing in the air.

OME, however, has a tendency to heal spontaneously with age, except in a small number of persistent cases. In the treatment of this disease, the surgical procedure should be adopted after careful observation of the clinical course, and the method of treatment may differ depending on age. As complete treatment or prevention of the disease is difficult at present, some palliative approaches should also be considered.

References

Bernstein JM, Okazaki T, Reisman RE (1976) Prostaglandins in middle ear effusions. Arch Otolaryngol 102:257–280

Bernstein JM, Praino MD, Neter E (1980) Detection of endotoxin in ear specimens from patients with chronic otitis media by means of the Limulus Amebocyte Lysate Test. Can J Micorbiol 26:645–646

Bluestone CD, Paradise JL, Beery QC (1972) Symposium on prophylaxis and treatment of middle ear effusion: IV. Physiology of the eustachian tube in the pathogenesis and management of middle ear effusions. Laryngoscope 82:1654–1670

Cantekin EI, Bluestone CD, Parkin LP (1976) Eustachian tube ventilatory function in children. Ann Otol Rhinol Laryngol 85 (Suppl 25):171–177

DeMaria TF, Briggs BR, Lim DJ, Okazaki N (1984) Experimental otitis media with effusion following middle ear inoculation of nonviable *H. influenzae*. Ann Oto Rhinol Laryngol 93:52–56

Dennis RG, Whitemire RN, Jackson RT (1976) Action of inflammatory mediators on middle ear mucosa. Arch Otolaryngol 102:420–424

Holmquist J, Renwall U (1974) Eustachian tube function in secretory otitis media. Arch Otolaryngol 99:59–61

Kawabata I, Nomura Y and Dohi T (1986) Middle ear pressure in patients with middle ear effusion—Direct measurement by pressure microtransducer. Auris Nasus Larynx 12 (Suppl 1):108–110

Kokko E (1974) Chronic secretory otitis media in children. A clinical study. Acta Otolaryngol Suppl 327:1–44

Liu YS, Lim DJ, Lang RW, Birck HG (1975) Chronic middle ear effusions: Immunological and bacteriological investigations. Arch Otolaryngol 101:278–286

Murphy D (1979) Negative pressure in the middle ear by ciliary propulsion of mucus through the eustachian tube. Laryngoscope 89:954–961

Nozoe T, Okazaki N, Koda Y, Ayani N, Kumazawa T (1984) Fluid clearance of the eustachian tube. In: Lim DJ (ed) Recent advances in otitis media with effusion. Decker Toronto, pp 66–68

Passali D, Bellussi L, Masieri S (1984) Transtympanic iontophoresis: Personal experience. Laryngoscope 94:802–806

Sato H, Takahashi H, Honjo I (1988) Transtympanic iontophoresis of dexamethasone and fosfomycin. Arch Otolaryngol 114:531–533

Senturia BH, Gessert CF, Carr CD, Baumann ES (1958) Studies concerned with tubotympanitis. Ann Otol Rhinol Laryngol 66:440–467

Silverstein H, Miller GF, Lindman RC (1966) Eustachian tube dysfunction as a cause for chronic secretory otitis in children. Laryngoscope 76:259–273

Takasaka T, Kaku Y, Shibahara Y, Hozawa K, Takeyama M, Kaneko Y, Kawamoto K (1984) Experimental otitis media with effusion: An immunoelectron microscopic study. In: Lim DJ (ed) Recent advances in otitis media with effusion Decker, Toronto, pp 88–91

Westergaard O (1970) Tubal function in patients with chronic secretory otitis media. Acta Otolaryngol 263:23–24

Chapter 6
Adenoid Vegetation and Otitis Media with Effusion

It is widely accepted that the adenoid vegetation, which occupies the nasopharynx, is closely related to the development and prognosis of otitis media with effusion (OME). Since Meyer's report on hearing improvement by adenoidectomy (1870), this surgical procedure has been routinely employed for the treatment of OME. The influence of the adenoids on OME may be explained by their relation to the eustachian tube or upper respiratory infection such as nasal sinusitis. However, the mechanisms by which the adenoids exert adverse effects on the middle ear have not been adequately elucidated.

On the other hand, questions have been raised recently on the therapeutic effects of adenoidectomy on OME (Rynnel-Dagöö 1978; Roydhouse 1980; Fiellau-Nikolajsen 1983), and among the opinions recommending surgery (Mackee 1963; Maw 1983; Bulman 1984) no consensus has been reached.

One of the causes of such a controversy is the fact the accurate evaluation of adenoid hypertrophy is rather difficult, either by the finger test or by lateral X-ray of the nasopharynx. For more reliable evaluation of the adenoids in relation to the eustachian tube, endoscopic examination of the nasopharynx was conducted in the study reported here. On the other hand, tests for objective evaluation of OME have not been fully established. In the present study, OME was evaluated primarily by pure-tone audiometry; tympanometry was employed as a supplementary test, because it has excessive sensitivity in some cases and is invalid except when the eardrum is intact.

Present questions to be answered in relation to the adenoids and the middle ear system are: (a) Do the adenoids have any mechanical influence on eustachian tube function? (b) is adenoidectomy effective for treatment of OME? and (c) does adenoidectomy relieve nasal sinusitis, which often complicates OME?

6.1 Adenoids and Eustachian Tube Function

Before investigating the relation between the adenoids and OME, the characteristics of the adenoids and eustachian tube were examined. Large adenoids that fill the nasopharyngeal space, as shown in Fig. 6.1, are likely to affect the patency of the eustachian tube since frequent obstruction of the pharyngeal orifice of

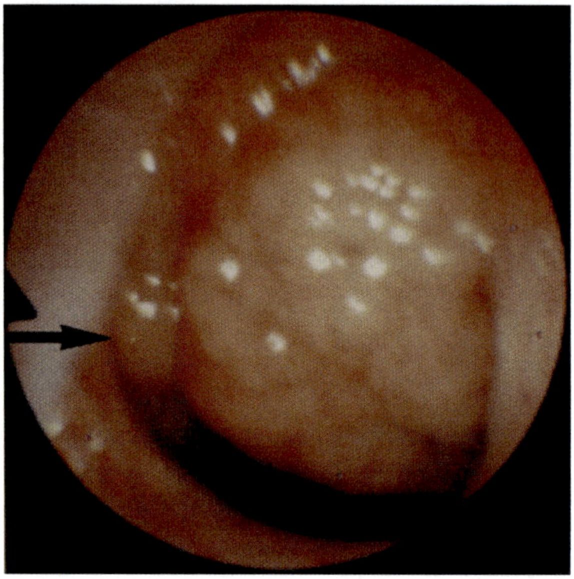

Fig. 6.1. Pharyngeal orifice of eustachian tube (*arrow*) compressed by enlarged adenoid

the eustachian tube by adenoid tissue was noted under endoscopic observation of the nasopharynx in OME patients (Honjo et al. 1982). There have been only a few studies (Bluestone et al. 1975; Tashima et al. 1986) as to whether the adenoids substantially impair eustachian tube function, particularly ventilatory function.

6.1.1 Impairment of Ventilation Function of Eustachian Tube by Adenoids

The adenoids were examined by endoscopy to determine whether adenoid tissue covers the pharyngeal orifice of the tube and exerts pressure upon it. The relation between these endoscopic findings and eustachian tube function was then tested both by the opening pressure and equilibration of the applied positive pressure upon swallowing.

Based on the endoscopic findings of the adenoids, 52 children with OME (aged 4–13 years) were divided into two groups: those with large adenoids obstructing the pharyngeal orifice of the tube, and those without such obstruction. The opening pressure of the tube was determined as described in Sect 4.1.1.1 by applying a certain positive pressure to the middle ear through the perforated eardrum, and the minimum pressure required for tubal opening was determined.

In the group with large adenoids, the mean opening pressure of the tube was 298 mmH_2O ($\pm$185 mmH_2O), while in the group with relatively small adenoids without tubal obstruction it was 307 mmH_2O ($\pm$187 mmH_2O); the difference between the two groups was not significant (Fig. 6.2). The frequency of normal opening pressure of the tube in each group was 79% and 74%, respectively.

These results indicate that large adenoids, which might exert pressure upon

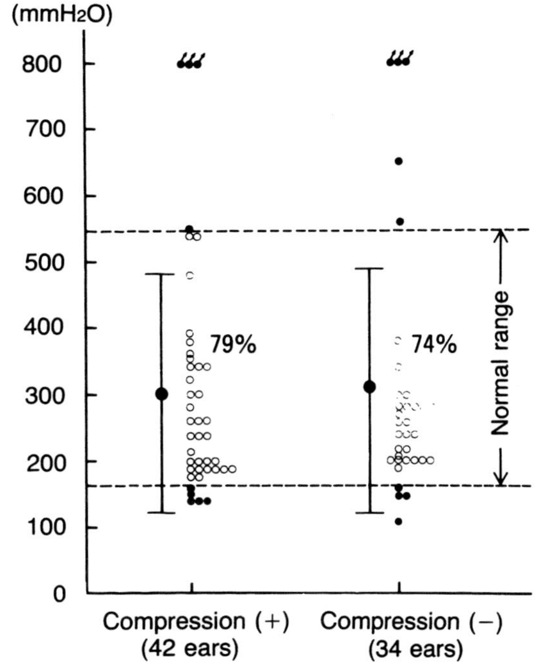

Fig. 6.2. Opening pressure of the tube in children with and without compression of the pharyngeal orifice by enlarged adenoids

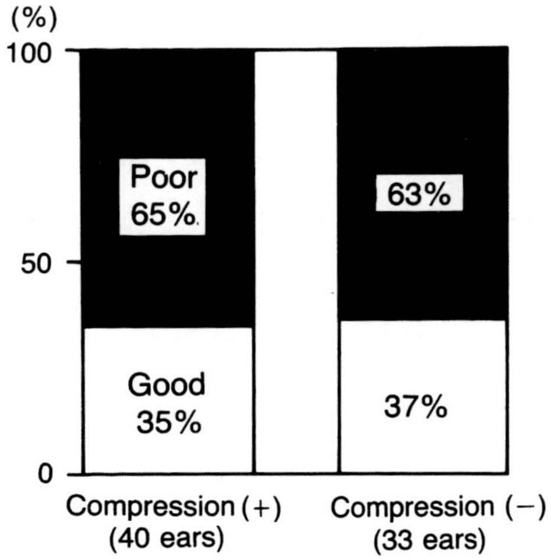

Fig. 6.3. Positive pressure test in children with and without enlarged adenoids by endoscopy

the pharyngeal orifice of the tube, do not necessarily affect the patency.

The dynamic function of the tube examined by the positive pressure test was good in 35% of the group with tubal obstruction by the adenoids and in 37% of the group without such obstruction (Fig. 6.3). The above examinations, which are mainly concerned with ventilatory function of the tube, revealed that the adenoids obstruct neither the pharyngeal orifice of the tube nor the eustachian tube itself.

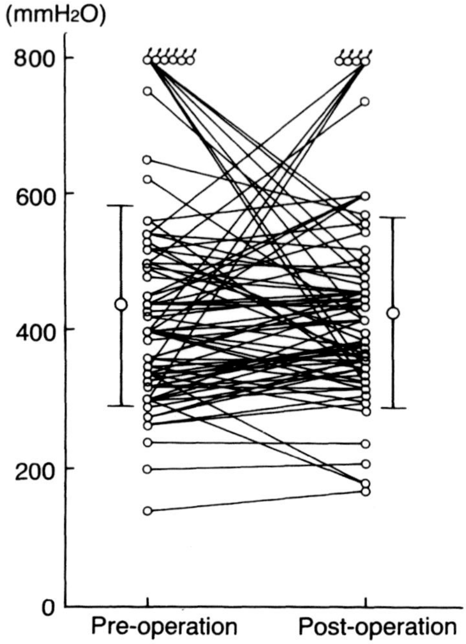

Fig. 6.4. Opening pressure of eustachian tube before and after adenoidectomy in 72 ears

6.1.2 Adenoidectomy and Improvement of Eustachian Tube Function

The effects of adenoidectomy on the eustachian tube were evaluated by examination of eustachian tube function before and immediately after adenoidectomy (short term), and for 6 months postoperatively (long term).

6.1.2.1 Short-Term Evaluation

Thirty-six children (aged 4–7 years) with OME who underwent adenoidectomy were examined under general anesthesia. The opening pressure of the eustachian tube was measured before and just after removal of the adenoids through the ventilation tube. Since the measurement was made in the supine position, the opening pressure was higher than that routinely measured in the sitting position.

The results showed that the mean opening pressure was 435 mmH_2O (± 154 mmH_2O) preoperatively and 429 mmH_2O (± 142 mmH_2O) postoperatively. However, this slight difference in the opening pressure was not significant (Fig. 6.4).

The present findings of short-term evaluation of the tube indicate that adenoids do not obstruct the eustachian tube, at least in the static condition.

6.1.2.2 Long-Term Evaluation

Next, the effects of adenoidectomy on the tubal function were examined for 6 months: 106 children (aged 5–7 years) with OME with adenoid vegetation were divided into two groups; 125 ears that underwent adenoidectomy with a ventilation tube (adenoidectomized group) and 60 ears with a ventilation tube alone

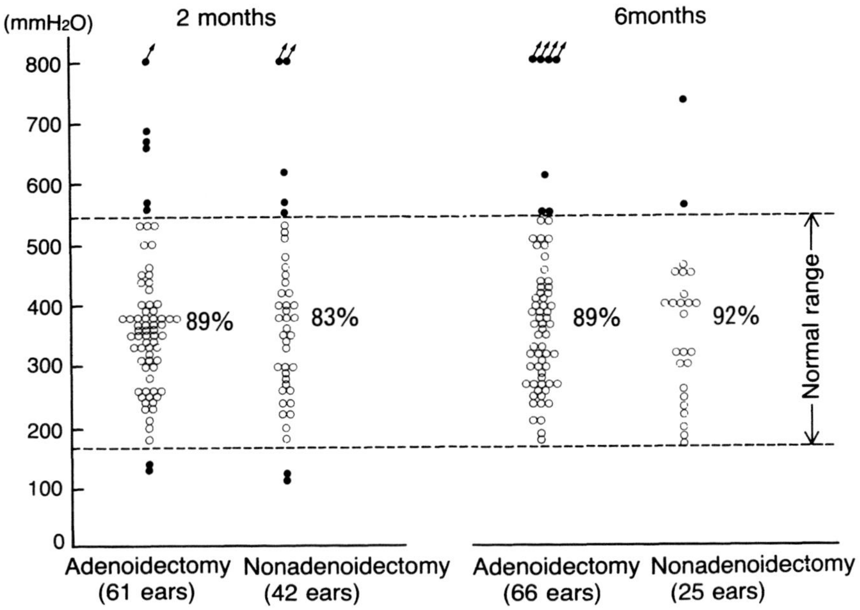

Fig. 6.5. Opening pressure of eustachian tube in children with and without adenoidectomy

(nonadenoidectomized group). Measurements of the opening pressure of the tube were made twice—at 2 months and 6 months after surgery.

In the adenoidectomized group, the mean opening pressure of the tube was 370 mmH_2O ($\pm$125 mmH_2O) and in the nonadenoidectomized group it was 374 mmH_2O ($\pm$157 mmH_2O) 2 months postoperatively; the values were 383 mmH_2O ($\pm$135 mmH_2O) and 359 mmH_2O ($\pm$128 mmH_2O) for the respective groups 6 months after surgery. At either examination, no significant differences in the opening pressure of the tube were noted between the two groups (Fig. 6.5). In both groups, the frequency of normal opening pressure of the tube was more than 80%. Therefore, even in the long-term observation, adenoidectomy has no significant effect on static ventilatory function of the eustachian tube.

These results indicate that adenoids do not exert any pressure on the pharyngeal orifice of the tube and that their surgical removal does not change the patency of the tube. It appears unlikely that large adenoids covering the pharyngeal orifice have no effect on the patency of the tube. However, considering the compliant nature of adenoid tissue, it may not affect the static condition of tubal patency.

On the other hand, the effects of adenoidectomy on the dynamic function of the eustachian tube were quite different. The results of the positive pressure test during swallowing were good in 53% of the adenoidectomized group, while only 32% of those in the nonadenoidectomized group showed normal values 1 week after the operation (Fig. 6.6), indicating significant improvement of the tubal

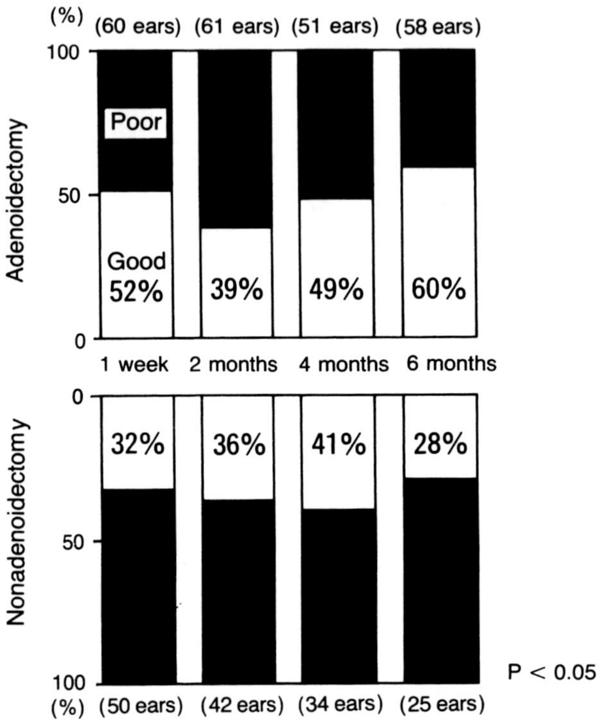

Fig. 6.6. Positive pressure test in children with and without adenoidectomy

function in the adenoidectomized group. The dynamic function of the eustachian tube in the adenoidectomized group was improved at 2 months and 4 months; 60% improvement was observed at 6 months after the surgery, while this was only 28% in the nonadenoidectomized (P<0.05). Although the results 1 week after surgery may include some effects of antibiotics used postoperatively, the subsequent improvements in the dynamic function of the tube are considered to be due to the surgical removal of the adenoid tissue. In the negative pressure test, however, the difference between the adenoidectomy and nonadenoidectomy groups was not significant, though the results were better in the first group at all points of time examined.

Tympanometry was carried out 6 months after adenoidectomy in 88 ears with intact eardrums in which the tympanostomy tube had become displaced. It was found that in the adenoidectomized group, tympanograms were of the A type in 47%, C type in 25%, and B type in 28% of cases, while they were of the A type in 30%, C type in 18%, and B type in 52% of cases in the nonadenoidectomized group. The type-B tympanogram, which indicates retention of fluid in the tympanic cavity, was significantly frequent (P<0.05) in the nonadenoidectomized group (Fig. 6.7). It was suggested that the disturbance of the middle ear was improved by normalization of the eustachian tube after adenoidectomy.

From these results, it is concluded that the dynamic function of the eustachian tube is improved by adenoidectomy.

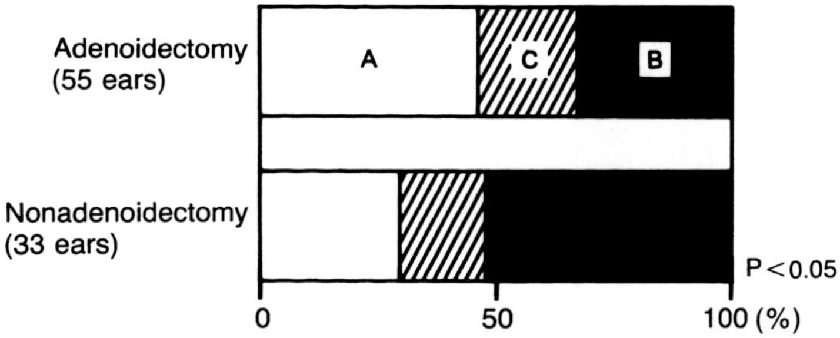

Fig. 6.7. Tympanograms in children with and without adenoidectomy

6.1.3 Summary

The mechanical effects of adenoid tissue on the eustachian tube were evaluated by ventilatory function tests in children with OME who underwent adenoidectomy and those who did not. The results were as follows.

a) Adenoids did not affect the opening pressure of the tube, indicating that they do not impair the static function.
b) The dynamic function of the tube during swallowing was improved significantly by adenoidectomy. The effect of surgery was also confirmed by the significant improvement in tympanometric findings.

6.2 Effects of Adenoidectomy on OME

The value of adenoidectomy, especially for treatment of OME in children, has been questioned by many investigators because this surgery is less effective for OME than was expected. The conclusion as to whether adenoidectomy is effective still remains controversial due to the difficulty of evaluating the effects. The factors that complicate analysis of the results are: (a) spontaneous recovery of OME with age; (b) reduction of the size of the adenoids with age; and (c) difficulty of objective evaluation of improvement in OME.

For these reasons, assessment of the effects of adenoidectomy was carried out in a relatively short period of 6 months in the present study. For evaluation of the condition of the ear, pure-tone audiometry was mainly used because it seemed to be more appropriate for this purpose than inspection of the eardrum or the tympanometric test.

6.2.1 Effectiveness of Adenoidectomy in OME

In 95 children with OME (5–7 years), 127 ears were divided into two groups according to the surgery they underwent. The first group consisted of 50 children who underwent adenoidectomy with insertion of a tympanostomy tube (adenoidectomy group, mean age 6.0 years), and the second group consisted of 45

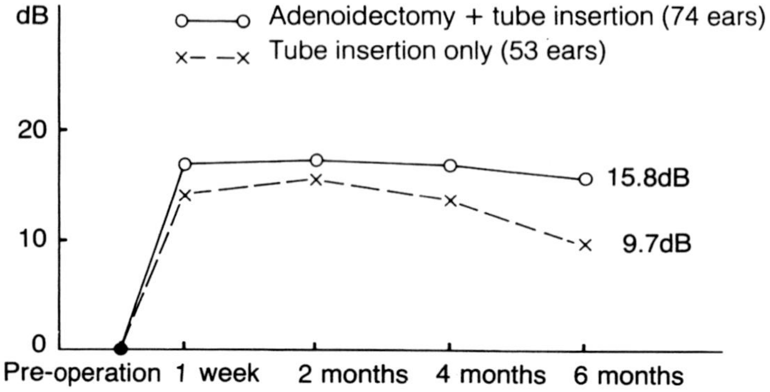

Fig. 6.8. Mean hearing gains in children with and without adenoidectomy

children who received insertion of the tube alone (nonadenoidectomy group, mean age 6.2 years).

Adenoidectomy was performed under general anesthesia, and insetion of a grommet-type tube in the eardrum was performed either simultaneously with adenoidectomy or separately under local anesthesia. Pure-tone audiometry was carried out before the operation as well as 1 week and 2, 4, and 6 months after. Hearing was evaluated by averaging three tones of 500 Hz, 1000 Hz and 2000 Hz.

In the adenoidectomized group, the mean hearing level of 29.5 dB improved immediately after operation, and the final hearing level at 6 months was 13.7 dB, with a total hearing gain of 15.8 dB. During the 6-month follow-up period, consistent improvement in hearing was noted (Fig. 6.8).

In the nonadenoidectomized group, on the other hand, the mean hearing level of 29.8 dB improved immediately after the tube insertion, owing to the removal of the middle ear fluid by myringotomy. However, the hearing began to worsen from 4 months, and the final gain of hearing at 6 months was 9.7 dB. The deterioration after 4 months was considered to be partly due to displacement of the tympanostomy tube (Fig. 6.8).

As the above observations were made randomly on two groups of children with OME, the effects of adenoidectomy judged by the hearing level may be obscured if the initial hearing was good enough in some cases or if it differed significantly between the two groups. In addition to this, previous observations included the effects of the tympanostomy tube as well as adenoidectomy, which may not be appropriate for exclusive evaluation of the role of adenoidectomy in the treatment of OME.

For more precise evaluation of the effect of adenoidectomy, therefore, comparisons were made among 55 selected ears that had an initial hearing loss of more than 20 dB and lost the tympanostomy tube at an early stage. In the adenoidectomy group (31 ears), the hearing showed marked improvement immediately after the operation but slightly worsened at 4–6 months (Fig. 6.9), probably due to the tympanostomy tube coming out. Despite this regression, the overall hearing gain after 6 months was 17.3 dB (Fig. 6.9). In the

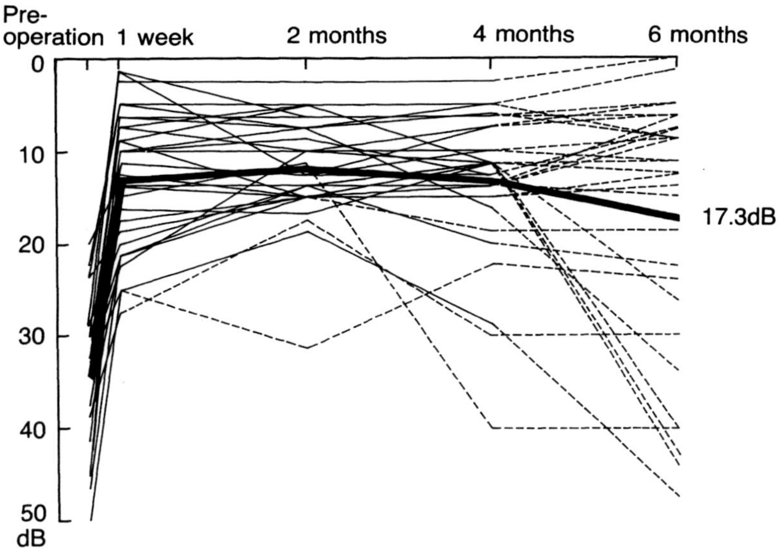

Fig. 6.9. Hearing levels in children with adenoidectomy in 30 ears. Preoperative hearing level > 20 dB. *Continuous line* tube was correctly in position, *broken line* tube was displaced

nonadenoidectomized group (24 ears), however, hearing improvement resulting from the insertion of the tube deteriorated markedly after 4 months, with only a 3.8 dB hearing gain at 6 months (Fig. 6.10). The difference in hearing improvement between the two groups, which were designed to be equal except for the factor of adenoidectomy, was 13.8 dB, indicating the marked effect of adenoidectomy (Fig. 6.11).

In general, the efficacy of a treatment should be evaluated after a long period of follow-up, but considering the tendency of spontaneous healing of OME in children, treatment that achieves quick and consistent effects is of more practical use. Though insertion of a tympanostomy tube has the advantage of a quick improvement in hearing, its consistency was not satisfactory in those patients whose tympanostomy tube were displaced.

The combined treatment of adenoidectomy with tube insertion permitted more satisfactory effects in speed and reliability on hearing improvement even in cases in which the tube came out. The significant difference between the results of the two methods of treatment, namely adenoidectomy plus tympanostomy tube and the tube insertion only, is considered to represent the effect of adenoidectomy on OME.

6.2.2 Summary

To examine the effect of adenoidectomy in the treatment of OME, the hearing level by pure-tone audiometry was followed up for 6 months in two groups of children with OME. It was found that those who underwent the combined ther-

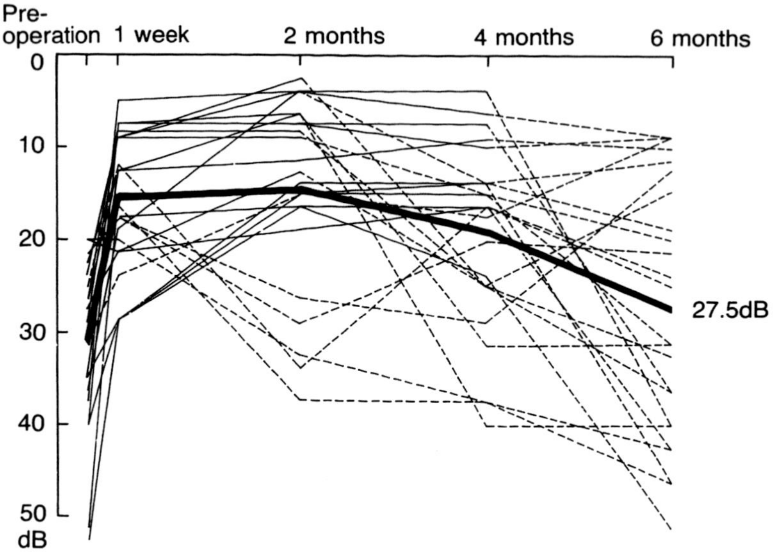

Fig. 6.10. Hearing levels in children without adenoidectomy in 24 ears. Preoperative hearing level > 20 dB. *Continuous line* tube was in position, *broken line* tube was displaced

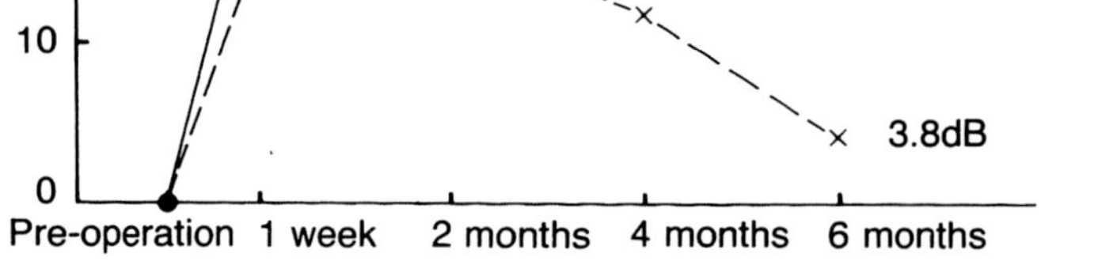

Fig. 6.11. Mean hearing gains in children with and without adenoidectomy. Preoperative hearing level > 20 dB. Tube was displaced

apies of adenoidectomy and insertion of a tympanostomy tube showed consistent improvement of hearing even when the tube became displaced. On the other hand, hearing in the nonadenoidectomized group deteriorated when the tube came out in the early stage, indicating the efficacy of adenoidectomy for OME.

6.3 Adenoidectomy and Nasal Sinusitis

Adenoids, which occupy the nasopharynx of children, are considered to affect the aerodynamics of the nose and nasopharynx. They also appear to be involved in the development and prolongation of inflammation in the nose and paranasal sinuses. The relation between nasal sinusitis and OME has been reported (Kowata 1980; Grote et al. 1980), and in our study 78% of the childen with OME were found to have nasal sinusitis, suggesting its etiological importance in OME. However, the effects of adenoidectomy on OME have not been studied with respect to nasal disease. Based on the hypothesis that the effect of adenoidectomy on OME is related to improvements in upper respiratory inflammation including nasal sinusitis, changes in nasal sinusitis after adenoidectomy were examined by roentgenography.

6.3.1 Effect of Adenoidectomy on Nasal Sinusitis

Seventy-eight children with OME (4–7 years) who had both large adenoids and nasal sinusitis were followed up for 6 months to 1 year. They were divided into two groups: 45 adenoidectomized children (mean age 5.9 years) and 33 nonadenoidectomized children (mean age 6.0 years). Nasal roentgenograms (occipitomental view) were taken twice before and 6 months to 1 year after adenoidectomy. Nasal sinusitis was classified into four grades according to the roentgenographic findings (Fig. 6.12), and judgment of improvement of the disease was made when two or more grades of improvement in the shadow of the paranasal sinuses were observed after adenoidectomy.

It was revealed that in the adenoidectomized group, nasal sinusitis was improved in 56% of cases, while in the nonadenoidectomized group only 24% showed improvement (Fig. 6.13). Significant improvements of nasal sinusitis in the adenoidectomized group ($P < 0.01$) indicated that this surgical procedure was effective for chronic inflammation in the nasopharynx and nasal sinuses.

6.3.2 Effect of Nasal Sinusitis on Eustachian Tube Function and Hearing

To clarify whether improvement of nasal sinusitis after adenoidectomy has any effect on eustachian tube function and on hearing, tubal function evaluated by

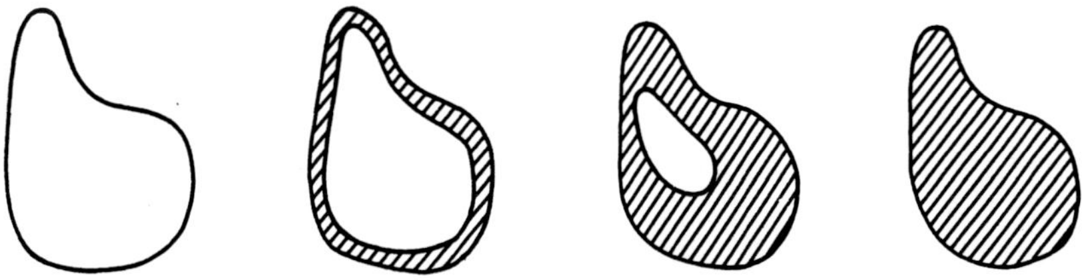

Fig. 6.12. Roentgenographic classification of findings in maxillary sinus

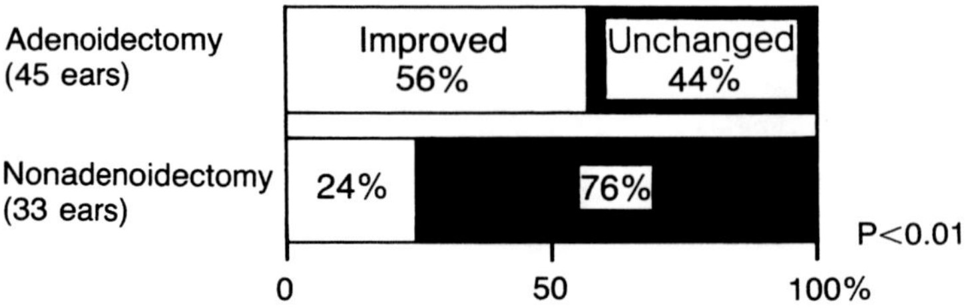

Fig. 6.13. Relation between adenoidectomy and improvement in nasal sinusitis

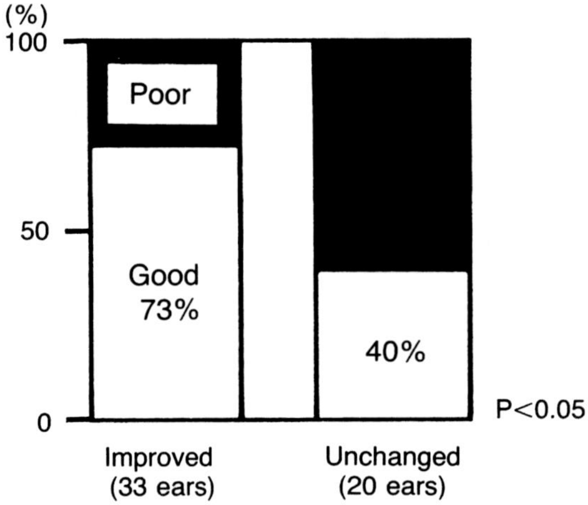

Fig. 6.14. Positive pressure test of the tube and improvement of nasal sinusitis in children with adenoidectomy

the positive pressure test and hearing by pure-tone audiometry were compared between two groups: 25 children with OME whose sinusitis was improved after the adenoidectomy, and 20 children who showed no improvement of sinusitis after the surgery.

The tubal function evaluated at 6 months by the positive pressure test was good in 73% of the OME children who had improved nasal sinusitis, but improvement of the tubal function was seen in only 40% of those with poor response to the surgery (Fig. 6.14). This indicated that the tubal function was significantly better ($P < 0.05$) when nasal sinusitis was improved by adenoidectomy.

Hearing improvement was evaluated in quite a small group of children with OME who showed a marked initial hearing loss of more than 20 dB. Nine ears with improvement in nasal sinusitis were found to have satisfactory hearing improvement (Fig. 6.15), while 16 ears with no improvement of sinusitis showed deteriorated hearing after tube displacement (Fig. 6.16). After 6 months, a marked difference of 15.1 dB was noted in the hearing between the two groups (Fig. 6.17).

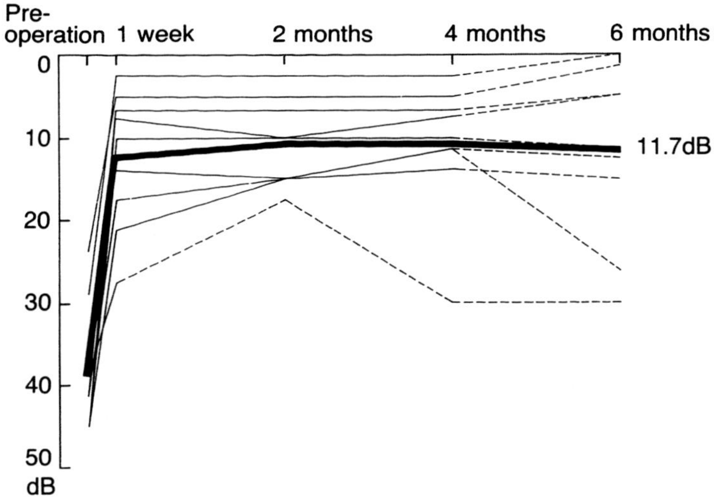

Fig. 6.15. Hearing levels in children with adenoidectomy in nine ears. Preoperative hearing level > 20 dB. Tube was displaced. Nasal sinusitis improved

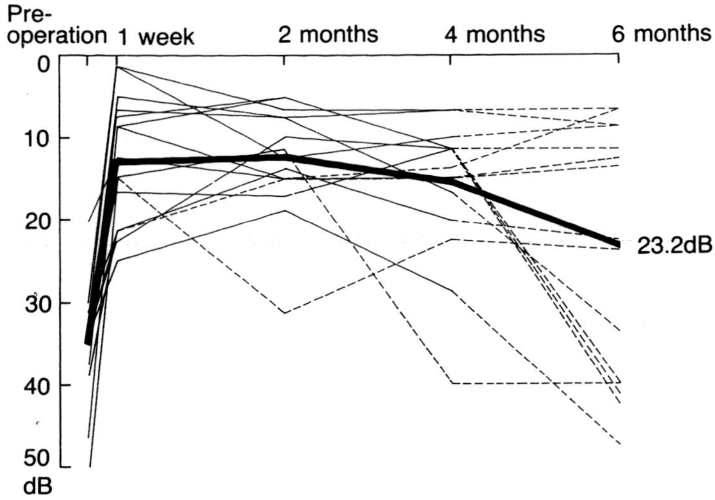

Fig. 6.16. Hearing levels in children with adenoidectomy in 16 ears. Preoperative hearing level > 20 dB. Tube was displaced. Nasal sinusitis unchanged

It was confirmed that among OME children who underwent adenoidectomy, those who had improved nasal sinusitis showed significant improvement both in tubal function and hearing compared with those who showed no improvement of the nose. Thus a certain process in which adenoidectomy improves the pathological condition of the eustachian tube via improvement of nasal sinusitis is suggested. However, the effects of adenoidectomy on the eustachian tube and

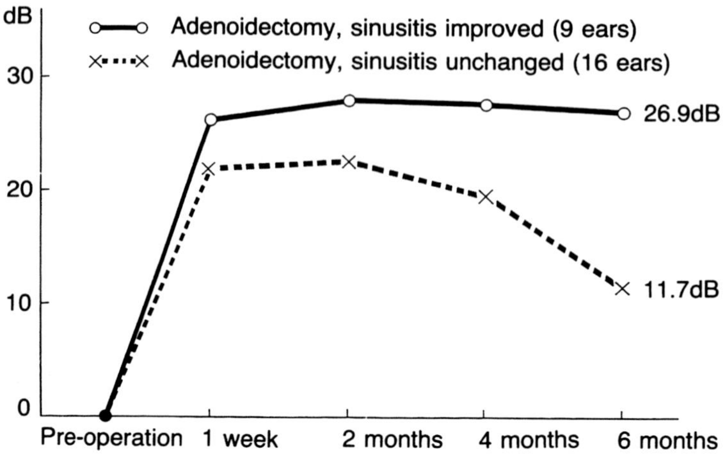

Fig. 6.17. Relation between mean hearing gains and improvement in nasal sinusitis in children with adenoidectomy

nasal sinusitis may be independent. At present, therefore, it is difficult to determine whether improvement of nasal sinusitis directly leads to improvement of the eustachian tube function or not.

6.3.3 Summary

By roentgenographic examination of 78 children who had both OME and nasal sinusitis, the effects of adenoidectomy on nasal sinusitis were examined. Since not only nasal sinusitis but eustachian tube function and hearing were also improved after the adenoidectomy concomitantly with remission of sinusitis, adenoidectomy was considered to cure OME partly via improvement of the pathological condition of the nasopharynx and paranasal sinusitis.

6.4 Summary of Chapter

The relation between the adenoids and the eustachian tube examined with respect of ventilation function of the tube revealed the absence of obstruction of the eustachian tube by the adenoids. This finding suggested that a large mass, which apparently obstructs the tubal orifice, exerts no significant pressure on the patency of the tube. However, the adenoids were found to impair the dynamic function of the tube during swallowing, and adenoidectomy improved this function of the tube significantly.

The efficacy of adenoidectomy for treatment of OME has been controversial, partly due to the late effects of the operation and partly to the rather subjective method of evaluation by inspecting the eardrum or the excessively sensitive method of tympanometry. When the effects of adenoidectomy on OME were evaluated according to hearing improvement, the surgical procedure was effective under every condition examined. However, such effects of adenoidectomy on OME cannot simply be attributed to improvements of the eustachian tube alone. Improvement of the tubal function secondary to improved nasal patency or nasal sinusitis by disappearance of either inflammation or the large mass in the nasopharynx might contribute to resolution of OME.

In any case, adenoidectomy has beneficial effects on children with OME. The operation, therefore, should be performed when its indications are justified by objective examination.

References

Bluestone CD, Cantekin EI, Beery QC (1975) Certain effects of adenoidectomy on eustachian tube ventilatory function. Laryngoscope 85:113–127

Bulman CH, Brook SJ, Beery MG (1984) A prospective randomized trial of adenoidectomy vs grommet insertion in the treatment of glue ear. Clin Otolaryngol 9:67–75

Fiellau-Nikolajsen M (1983) Tympanometry and secretory otitis media. Acta Otolaryngol (Suppl) 394:1–73

Grote JJ, Kuijpers W (1980) Middle ear effusion and sinusitis. J Laryngol Otol 94:177–183

Honjo I, Ushiro K, Haji T (1982) Pharyngeal orifice of the eustachian tube in otitis media with effusion. Jibi Inkoka 54:880–886 (in Japanese with English abstract)

Kowata I (1980) Pediatric otitis media and sinusitis. Jibi Inkoka 52:559–566 (in Japanese with English abstract)

Mackee WJE (1963) A controlled study of the effects of tonsillectomy and adenoidectomy in children. J Prev Soc Med 17:49–69

Maw AR (1983) Chronic otitis media with effusion (glue ear) and adenotonsillectomy: Prospective randomized controlled study. Br Med J 287:1586–1588

Meyer W (1870) On adenoid vegetations in the nasopharyngeal cavity. Med Surg Trans (London) 53:191–215

Roydhouse N (1980) Adenoidectomy for otitis media with mucoid effusion. Ann Otol Rhinol Laryngol 89 (Suppl 68): 312–315

Rynnel-Dagöö B (1978) Effects of adenoidectomy: A controlled two-year follow-up. Ann Otol Rhinol Laryngol 87:272–278

Tashima K, Mitoma T, Hamada E, Honjo I (1986) Effect of adenoidectomy on hearing of children with otitis media with effusion. Pract Otol (Kyoto) 79:557–564 (in Japanese with English abstract)

Chapter 7
Nasopharyngeal Carcinoma and Otitis Media with Effusion

Nasopharyngeal carcinoma (NPC) often accompanies otitis media with effusion (OME) and is closely related to the middle ear disease via the eustachian tube. The frequency of ear disease in NPC patients ranges from 25% to 50% (Godtfredsen et al. 1965; Sawaki 1979; Dickson 1981), but OME may be the only primary manifestation of NPC in some patients. It is important for otolaryngologists, therefore, to remember the association between these two disorders. On the other hand, the manner in which OME develops in patients with NPC has not been clarified. Such knowledge may contribute to understanding the role of the eustachian tube in the development of middle ear disease in general.

The questions to be answered in this chapter are: (a) What are the characteristics of eustachian tube disorders in NPC patients? (b) what are the differences between OME in patients with and without NPC? and (c) is there a relation between progression of nasopharyngeal carcinoma and disorders of the eustachian tube?

Patients with NPC in our clinic and in the Department of Otolaryngology, National Taiwan University were examined by endoscopy of the nasopharynx, computed tomography (CT) scan, and magnetic resonance imaging (MRI).

7.1 Ear Symptoms of NPC

A sensation of compression in the ear and hearing impairment are frequent symptoms at the early stage of NPC. Partly due to the rareness of NPC, however, patients with these symptoms may be regarded as simply having stenosis of the eustachian tube or OME and treated only by myringotomy or insertion of a tympanostomy tube, leading to a delay of proper treatment. Therefore, the significance of ear symptoms with respect to diagnosis, treatment, and prognosis of NPC were reexamined in 27 patients with NPC (13 males and 9 females, mean age 55.7 years) admitted to our department between 1975 and 1986.

7.1.1 Initial Symptoms of NPC

The symptoms that accompany NPC were divided into three categories: a mass of the neck (37.1%), ear symptoms (33.3%), and nasal symptoms (29.6%; Fig.

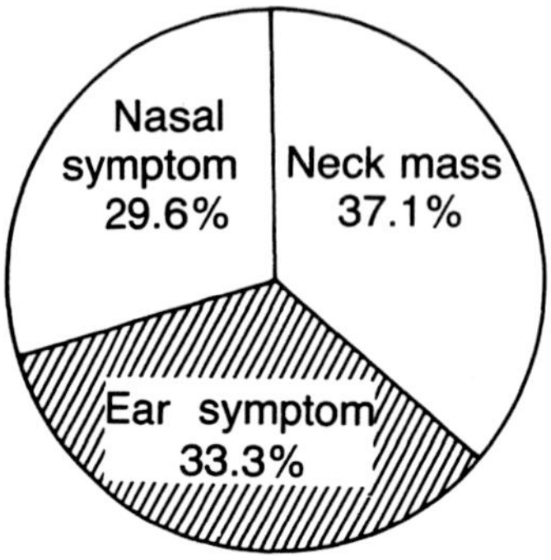

Fig. 7.1. Initial symptoms of NPC

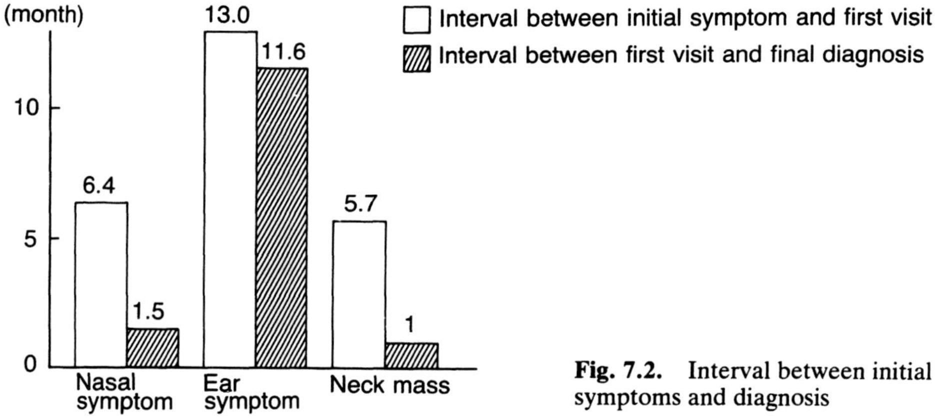

Fig. 7.2. Interval between initial symptoms and diagnosis

7.1). Ear symptoms such as hearing impairment or sensation of fullness in the ear, which are often associated with OME, occurred frequently next to a mass in the neck region. The frequency of ear symptoms varies with different reports, but hearing impairment and the sensation of ear fullness should not be overlooked as an initial sign of NPC.

7.1.2 Interval Between Onset of Symptoms and Diagnosis of NPC

Most patients referred to us from other physicians were already suspected of having NPC. However, the mean interval between the onset of the initial symptoms and their first visit to a doctor was significantly longer (13.0 months) when the symptoms were related to the ear than with symptoms of a mass in the neck (5.7 months) or of the nose (6.4 months; Fig. 7.2). Moreover, the period between the first visit to a doctor and diagnosis of NPC was 11.6 months in patients with ear symptoms, in contrast to 1 month in those with a mass of the neck or 1.5 months in those with nasal symptoms.

The delay in diagnosis in patients with ear symptoms may be partly due to the patient's attitude in regarding them as less important than neck masses, and also to the doctor mistaking such symptoms as OME or simply stenosis of the eustachian tube.

Table 7.1. Relation between initial symptoms and TN classification

N \ T	1	2	3	4	Total
0		○ ○		○ ○	0%
1			●	○ ● ● ● ●	83.3%
2		○ ● ● ●	○ ●		66.7%
3	○				0%
Total	0%	50%	66.7%	57.1%	

T tumor, *N* lymph node, ○ nasal symptoms, ● ear symptoms

7.1.3 Initial Symptoms with TN Classification and 5-Year Survival Rate

Concerning the TN (tumor, lymph node) classification, NPC tended to be more advanced in patients with ear symptoms than in those with nasal symptoms (Table 7.1), indicating a delay in detecting NPC when the initial sign was related to the ear.

The 5-year survival rate in our department was 35% for all patients with NPC. When viewed from the initial sign, the survival rate in those with a mass in the neck region was 15%, followed by 28% in those with ear symptoms. The poor prognosis associated with neck metastases may be related to extension of the tumor from the primary lesion, but the almost equal survival rate in patients with ear symptoms is considered to be due to the delay in the diagnosis of NPC.

7.1.4 Summary

The following results were obtained by examination of 27 patients with NPC.

a) About one-third of the patients showed ear symptoms as the initial manifestation of NPC, and they tended to be diagnosed as having only OME or stenosis of the eustachian tube.
b) NPC with initial symptoms in the ear required a longer period for diagnosis, and the 5-year survival rate was lower than in patients who showed nasal symptoms as the initial sign of NPC.

7.2 Eustachian Tube Function in Patients with NPC

OME in NPC patients is considered to be caused by impairment of eustachian tube function. However, we have no knowledge on the nature or degree of eustachian tube disorders in NPC. In this study, an examination was made of how the eustachian tube is affected by progression of the tumor in 60 previously untreated patients (113 ears) with different stages of NPC (male to female ratio 1.73:1, mean age 49.3 years). Tumors were histologically classified according to

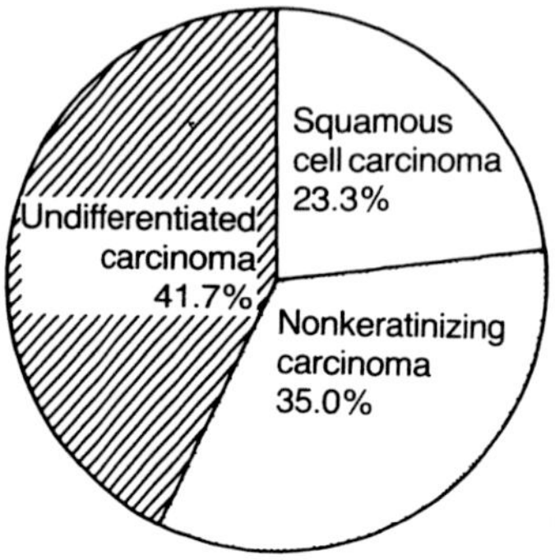

Fig. 7.3. Histological classification of NPC (60 cases)

the WHO system. Epidermoid carcinoma was included in the squamous cell carcinoma in this study. The poorly differentiated type of tumor was found most frequently (Fig. 7.3).

Eustachian Tube function was evaluated with respect to ventilatory function (opening pressure, positive and negative pressure tests) and clearance function through the perforated eardrum. Myringotomy of the asymptomatic ear was performed with the consent of the patient.

7.2.1 Eustachian Tube Impairment in NPC

Eustachian Tube function was evaluated in terms of its relation to the tumor in the nasopharynx and the presence of OME. According to the findings obtained by endoscopy in the nasopharynx and otoscopy in the eardrum, NPC patients were divided into the following three groups (when the tumor involved both ears, each ear was regarded as being on the tumor side): Group 1 (35 ears), OME on the tumor side; group 2 (55 ears), no OME on the tumor side; group 3 (23 ears), no OME on the non-tumor side.

In group 1, the opening pressure of the eustachian tube was within the normal range in 65.7% of subjects, but it was high in 28.6%, with extremely high values of more than 800 mmH_2O (off the scale) in 20.0% (Fig. 7.4). The results of the positive pressure test during swallowing were good in only 17.1% of subjects. In the negative pressure test, 97.1% of the subjects showed impaired function. The clearance function of the tube in the dye test was good in 37.5% of subjects, but poor in 62.5%, with no dye elimination (off the scale) in 50%. Both opening pressure of the tube and clearance time were off the scale in 14.3% of subjects in group 1, which indicated organic obstruction of the eustachian tube.

In group 2, the opening pressure of the tube was within the normal range in 70.9% of subjects, but high in 18.2%, with 9.1% of the values being extremely high (Fig. 7.5). The results of the positive pressure test during swallowing were good in 60.0% of subjects, while those of the negative pressure test were good in 41.8%. The clearance function of the tube was normal in 87.0% of subjects, but delayed in 13.0%, with 7.4% showing no elimination of the dye.

In group 3, the opening pressure of the tube was normal in 78.3% of subjects and did not exceed 800 mmH_2O in any of the ears (Fig. 7.6). The positive pres-

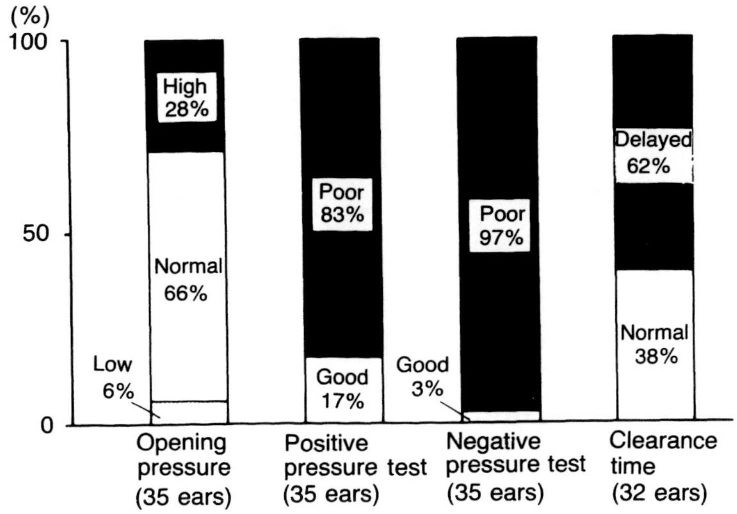

Fig. 7.4. Eustachian tube function in group 1 (tumor side with OME; 35 ears)

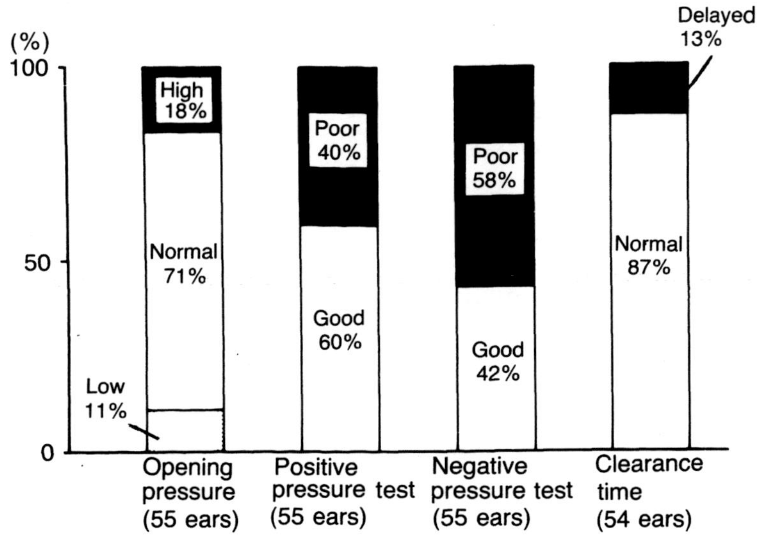

Fig. 7.5. Eustachian tube function in group 2 (tumor side without OME; 55 ears)

sure test showed good results in 87.0% of subjects, while the negative pressure test showed good results in 78.3%. The clearance function of the tube was normal in 91.0% of subjects, but it was delayed in 9.0%, with 4.5% showing no dye elimination.

The ears on the side without NPC were completely free of any disease such as OME, and the opening pressure, dynamic ventilatory function, and clearance

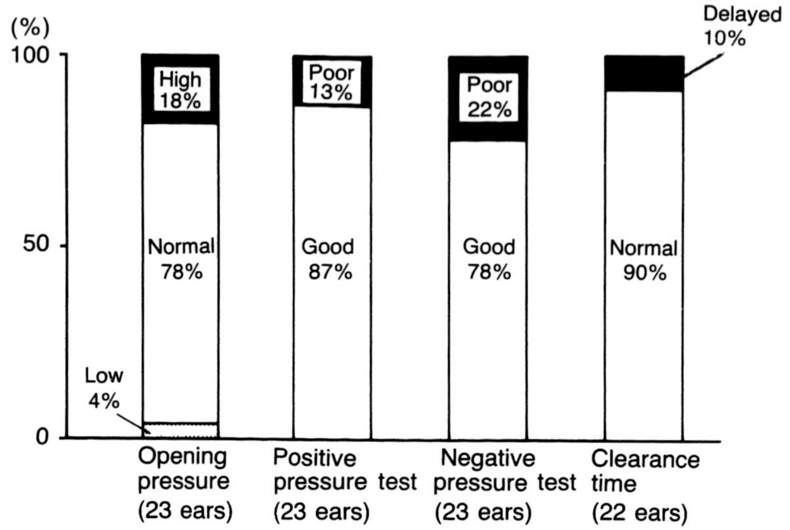

Fig. 7.6. Eustachian tube function in group 3 (non-tumor side without OME; 23 ears)

function of the eustachian tube were normal in more than 78% of these ears. These results indicate that before they were affected by NPC, the ears on the tumor side had normal function of the eustachian tube.

7.2.2 NPC and Eustachian Tube Function

The opening pressure, an index of organic stenosis of the eustachian tube, showed no significant difference among the ears on the tumor side with OME (group 1), those on the tumor side without OME (group 2), and those on the non-tumor side without OME (group 3; Fig. 7.7). This indicates that NPC exerts little compression on the eustachian tube, which may lead to OME.

With respect to the dynamic functions of the tube during swallowing, the results of the positive pressure test were poor in 82.9% of the subjects in group 1 with OME, which was significantly worse than the other two groups without OME (Fig. 7.8). Differences in the results of the positive pressure test depending on the presence of OME indicate a close relation between the dynamic function of the tube and development of OME on the side with NPC.

The results of the negative pressure test in the OME group were poorer (97.1%) than those (58.2%) in group 2 without OME even on the tumor side. However, between the two groups without OME, the results were significantly worse in group 2 than in group 3 (Fig. 7.8). These poor results in the negative pressure test before any manifestation of ear disease indicate that the ability to relieve negative middle ear pressure during swallowing is the first to be impaired in patients with NPC. As OME is absent in this period, OME is unlikely to arise from impairment of dynamic function of the tube alone. This finding is in close agreement with the condition of eustachian tube dysfunction observed in the

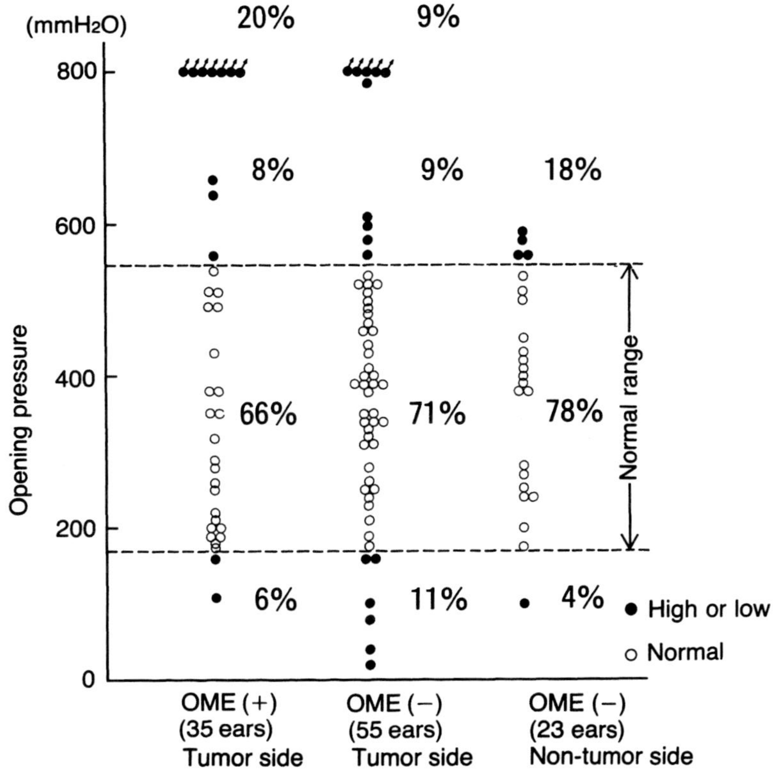

Fig. 7.7. Opening pressure of tube in NPC patients. No significant difference was found among the three groups

convalescent stage of children with OME. From these observations, impaired function to relieve negative pressure during swallowing is considered to be a necessary condition in the development of OME both in NPC and non-NPC patients.

The clearance function of the eustachian tube was significantly impaired in group 1 with OME as compared with groups 2 and 3 with no OME (Fig. 7.9). Since the patency of the tube was relatively intact in each group with NPC, this impaired clearance function was considered to depend largely on impairment of ciliary activity in the tube. These findings were consistent with those in non-NPC adults with OME in that relief of negative pressure was very poor, followed by impaired clearance function, and opening pressure of the tube was almost normal. Even in the ears on the affected side, only 13% of the cases showed both abnormally high opening pressure and delayed clearance of the tube, indicating infrequent organic obstruction of the eustachian tube by NPC. This observation was consistent with the report that NPC involving the cartilagenous and bony tissue rarely damaged the mucosa of the eustachian tube (Druss 1940).

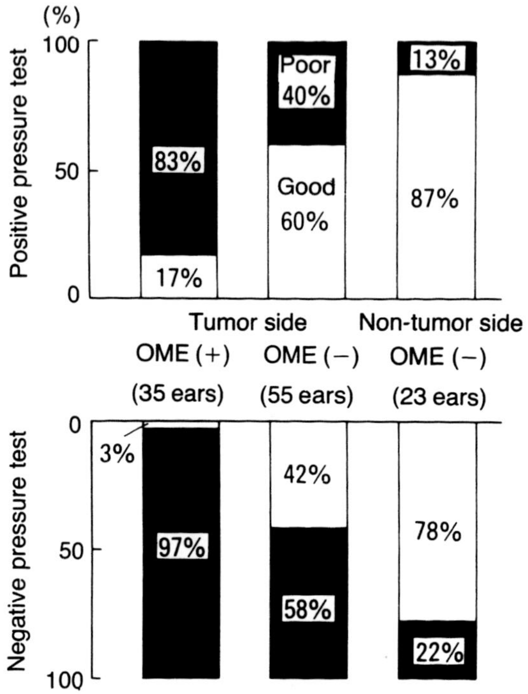

Fig. 7.8. Dynamic functions of tube in NPC patients. Significant differences were found among the three groups

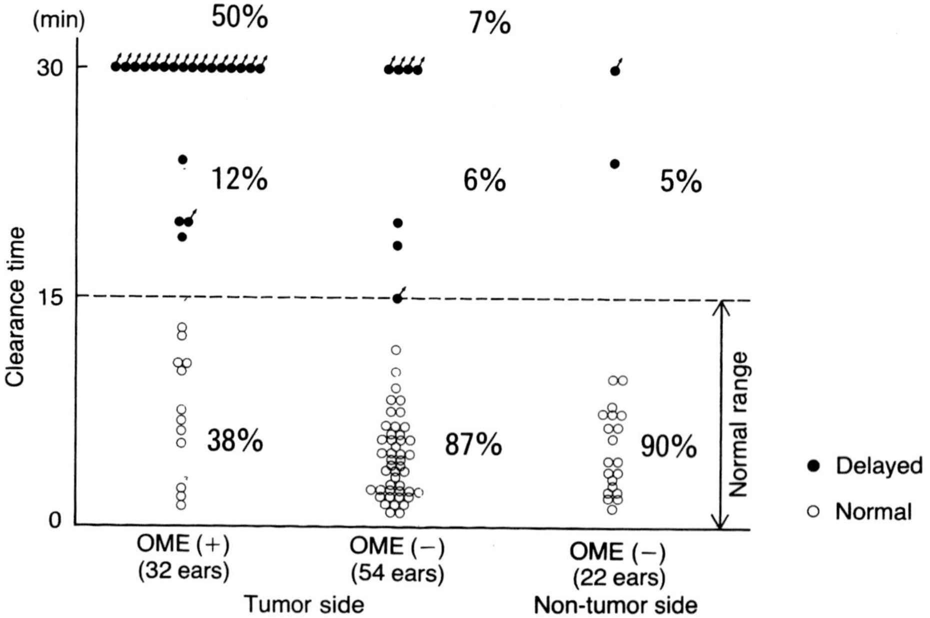

Fig. 7.9. Clearance function of tube in patients with NPC. Clearance function in group 1 was significantly worse than in groups 2 and 3

7.2.3 Summary

Examination of the eustachian tube in 113 ears of patients with NPC showed the following.

a) Abnormally high pressure for tubal opening was observed only in 13% of all the ears of patients with NPC, suggesting that mechanical obstruction of the tube is not a primary factor in the development of OME in these patients.
b) Ears with OME showed an almost total loss of negative pressure equalization by swallowing, indicating a pathological condition of the tube similar to that of OME without NPC.
c) Impairment of clearance function of the tube was closely related to OME, suggesting the involvement of inflammation, which impairs ciliary activity of the tube, in the development of OME.

From these observations, organic obstruction of the tube does not appear to be responsible for the development of OME in patients with NPC. Both impairment of dynamic tubal function and inflammation producing effusion were presumed to be the factors causing OME in NPC patients.

7.3 Inflammatory Factors in NPC

To clarify inflammatory factors in OME of NPC patients, prostaglandin E_2 (PGE_2) levels in the effusion of 14 ears in 13 NPC patients were measured.

7.3.1 PGE_2 in Middle Ear Effusion of NPC

The effusion was serous in ten and mucous in three ears. The PGE_2 level was 126–2475 pg/ml (1008 ± 847.6 pg/ml; Fig. 7.10), which is 15–295 times higher than the normal serum level. The mean value of PGE_2 in NPC patients was significantly higher than that of non-NPC adults with OME (serous in 16 and mucous in two).

PGE_2 is known to be closely related to inflammatory reactions and to be a useful indicator of inflammation. The present finding of high PGE_2 concentrations in the effusion suggested that inflammation is more severe in OME of NPC than in OME of non-NPC.

In patients with NPC, inflammation around the tumor (Teoh 1957; Thomas et al. 1984) and production of inflammatory agents from tumor cells (Panje 1981) have been reported. The present finding of high PGE_2 levels in NPC patients is in agreement with these reports.

7.3.2 Summary

Examination of PGE_2 levels in the effusion of NPC patients showed the following.

a) The PGE_2 level in the middle ear effusion of NPC patients was higher than the normal serum level.
b) The PGE_2 level was also significantly higher than that in non-NPC adult patients with OME.

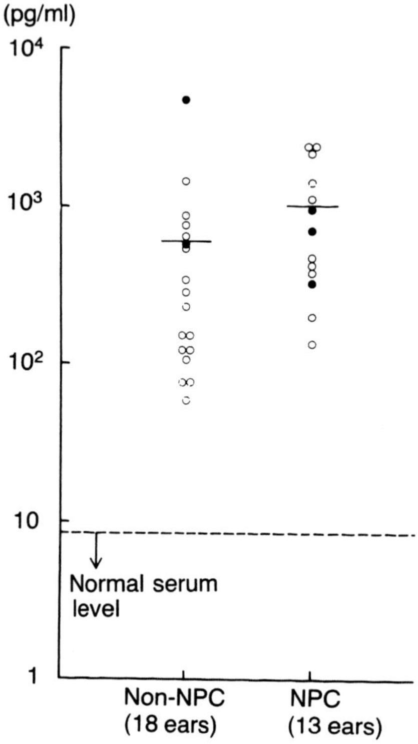

Fig. 7.10. PGE_2 in middle ear effusion. PGE_2 values in NPC patients were significantly higher than in non-NPC adult patients with OME

These results suggest that OME in NPC patients is related to inflammation induced by the nasopharyngeal tumor.

7.4 CT Findings and Eustachian Tube Function

The pathogenesis of OME in NPC patients has been considered to be eustachian tube dysfunction due to the tumor extension around the tube. However, the tumor size, site, or extension around the eustachian tube in relation to either the tubal function or OME remain to be elucidated. To clarify these relations, examination of NPC by CT scan, which permits observation of the deep part of the tube, and tests of tubal functions were carried out in 70 ears of 37 patients with NPC. Tumor staging based on CT findings of the tumor around eustachian tube is as follows:

Stage 0—no tumor
Stage 1—tumor does not occupy Rosenmüller's fossa
Stage 2—tumor occupies Rosenmüller's fossa
Stage 3—tumor compresses parapharyngeal space (low-density area)
Stage 4—tumor occupies parapharyngeal space

Representative CT scans for each grade are also presented in Fig. 7.11.

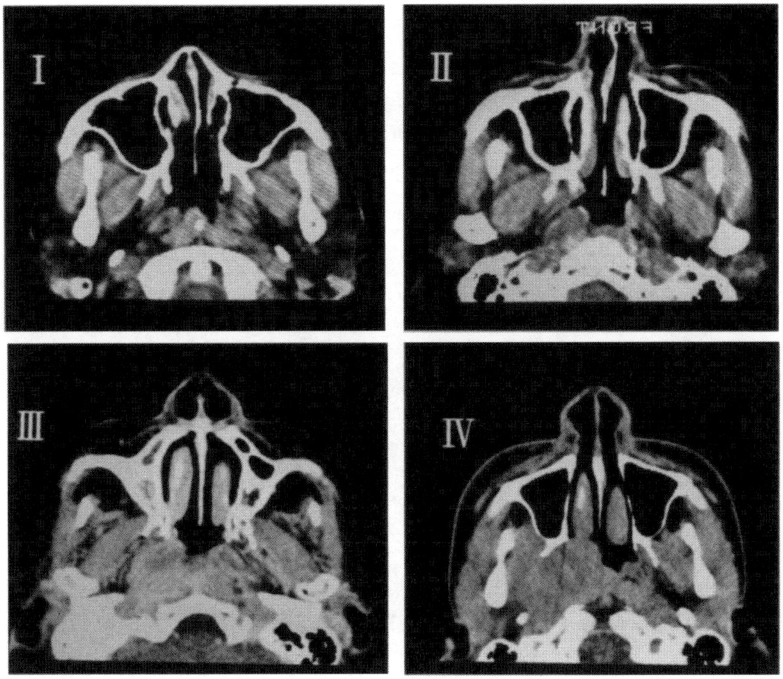

Fig. 7.11. CT finding at each stage

7.4.1 Eustachian Tube Function and Tumor Progression by CT Scan

The relation between the opening pressure of the tube and degree of the tumor by CT scan was studied (Fig. 7.12). Impairment of opening pressure of the tube was within 17% until the tumor extension of stage 3, in which the fatty tissue of the parapharyngeal space is compressed. The tubal function was first impaired in more than half of the cases, with the tumor invading the parapharyngeal space (stage 4). Thus, it was suggested that the patency of the tube was infrequently affected in NPC patients as in non-NPC patients.

Dynamic function of the tube as assessed by the positive and negative pressure tests was impaired in proportion to the progression of the tumor judged by CT scan (Fig. 7.13). The results of the negative pressure test, in particular, were poor in more than 20% of patients, even in those at stage 0 where no tumor was detected by CT. On the other hand, the positive pressure test showed impairment in about half the subjects when the tumor reached stage 3, which affects the parapharyngeal space. Thus, relief of the negative pressure was considered to be more affected than that of positive pressure.

The ventilatory function of the tube in relation to the stage of tumor evaluated by CT indicated that invasion of the tumor toward the parapharyngeal space around the eustachian tube impairs tubal function. The poor results of the negative pressure test suggest that the ability to relieve negative middle ear pressure

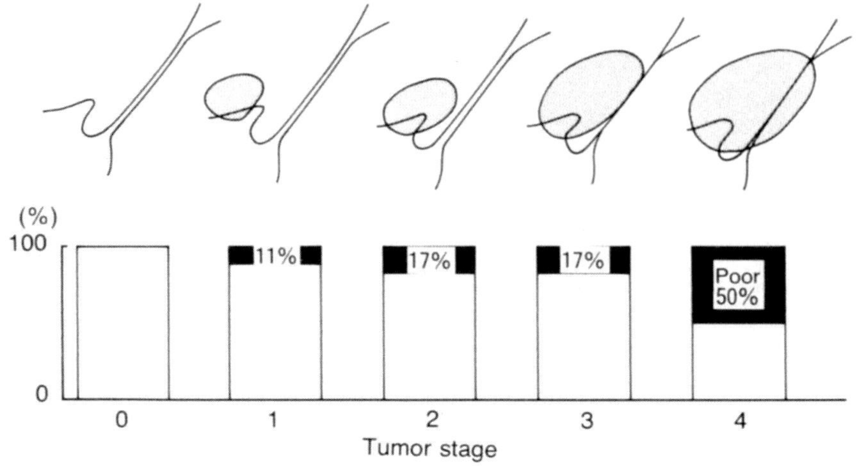

Fig. 7.12. Tumor stage and opening pressure of tube

during swallowing is also most vulnerable in NPC patients. However, the opening pressure of the tube was not impaired unless the tumor had invaded laterally to fill the parapharyngeal space. Therefore, it is not simple occlusion of the tube by the tumor, but impairment of dynamic function of the tube during swallowing appears to be most important in the development of OME in NPC patients.

The clearance function was first impaired when the tumor had progressed to stage 4 to fill the parapharyngeal space. Thus, the ciliary activity of the eustachian tube remained within the normal range until the tumor had invaded extensively.

7.4.2 Incidence of OME in NPC

The incidence of OME increased proportionally with progression of the tumor judged by the CT scan. The incidence exceeded 50% in NPC patients with stage 3, showing a rapid increase of OME after involvement of the parapharyngeal space by the tumor (Fig. 7.14).

7.4.3 Relation Between Degree of Tumor and Impairment of Eustachian Tube

Impairment of the eustachian tube and OME was viewed in relation to the progression of the tumor by CT scan. With progression of the tumor from stages 0 to 4, the ability to relieve negative pressure, the ability to relieve positive pressure, clearance function, and opening pressure of the tube deteriorated in this order. Thus, it was demonstrated that the relief of negative pressure was the most affected, whereas the opening pressure was the least influenced by the carcinoma around the eustachian tube. The incidence of OME correlated with the impairment of any tubal function, but most closely with the impairment of clearance function of the tube (Fig. 7.15).

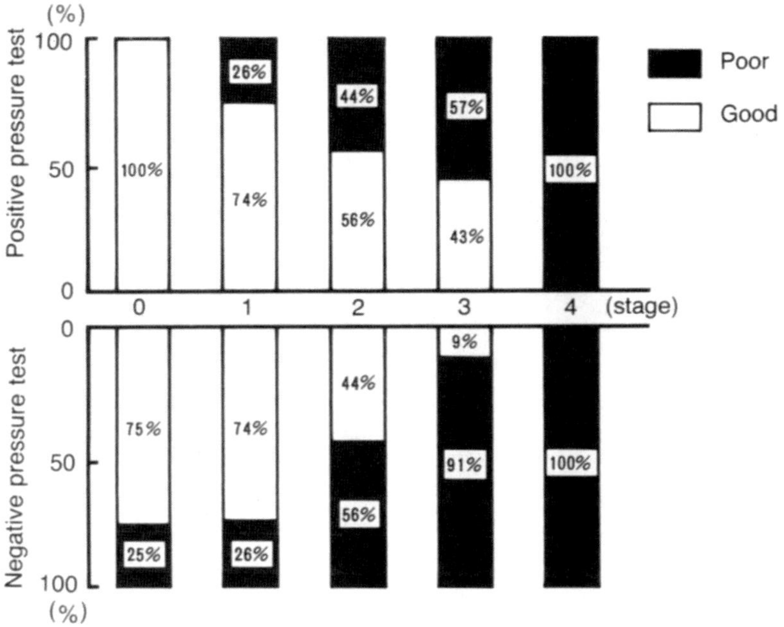

Fig. 7.13. Tumor stage and dynamic function of tube

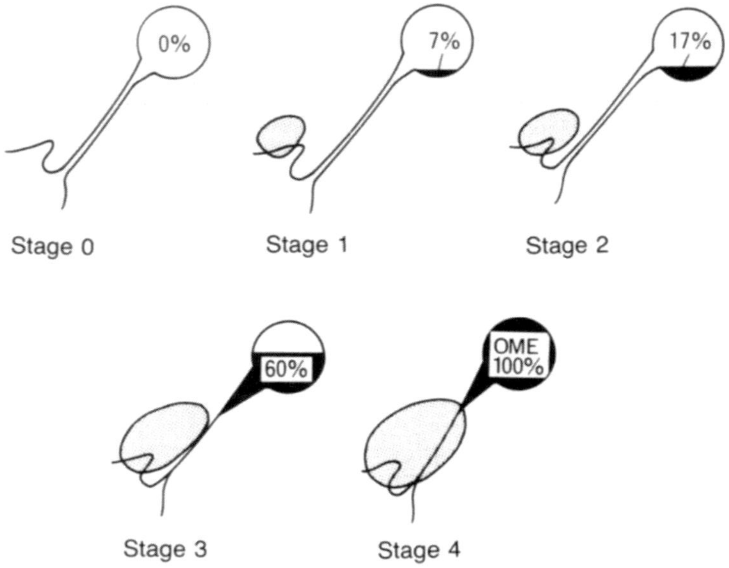

Fig. 7.14. Tumor stage and incidence of OME

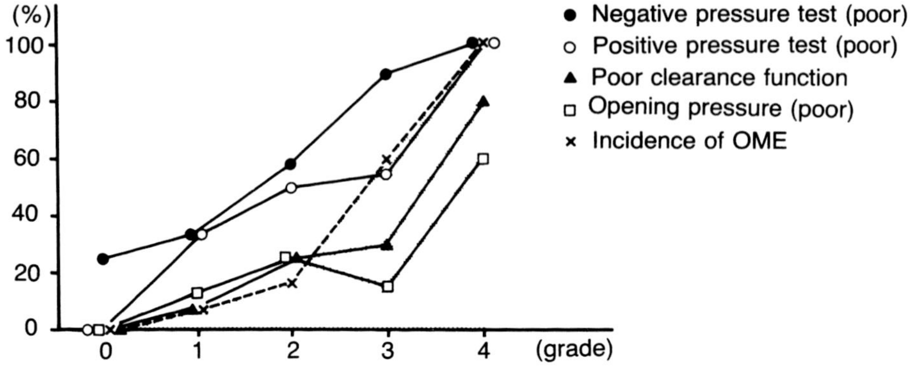

Fig. 7.15. Relation between tumor stage, eustachian tube function, and incidence of OME

7.4.4 Summary

With lateral progression of NPC toward the pharyngeal orifice of the tube and the parapharyngeal space, both the incidence of OME and impairment of the eustachian tube increased. Impairment of the tubal functions in NPC patients took place in the following order: the ability to relieve negative middle ear pressure, the ability to relieve positive middle ear pressure, clearance function, and opening pressure.

7.5 Magnetic Resonance Imaging in NPC

An association between the progression of NPC and OME was demonstrated by CT scan. Magnetic resonance imaging (MRI), which has come into clinical use in recent years, was considered as a mean of further elucidating the relation because it gives higher soft tissue resolution than conventional CT.

The MRI system used was a model with a 1.5-T superconduction magnet, and tomograms were obtained along the base line that passed through both the upper ends of the external ear canal and the tips of the first upper incisors, which is parallel to the eustachian tube. The thickness of the section was 3.0 mm, and the interval between the sections was 1.5 mm. Images were obtained using a 30-cm headcoil with a pixel size of 0.94 × 0.94 mm. The pulse sequence was spin-echo: repetition time (TR) 2000 ms; echo time (TE) 40, 80 ms.

Nineteen normal individuals were used as controls. In the controls, a linear low-signal area corresponding to the tubal cartilage was observed in the upper eustachian tube where it comes into contact with the skull base, and a high-signal area corresponding to the tubal mucosa was identified lateral to the cartilage (Fig. 7.16a). A linear low-signal area of the tubal cartilage was observed clearly also in a lower section (Fig. 7.16b). In the image lower than the section in Fig. 7.16b (Fig. 7.17a), the tubal cartilage disappeared and the tensor and levator muscles were seen to be separated by a high signal layer of fat tissue. The levator

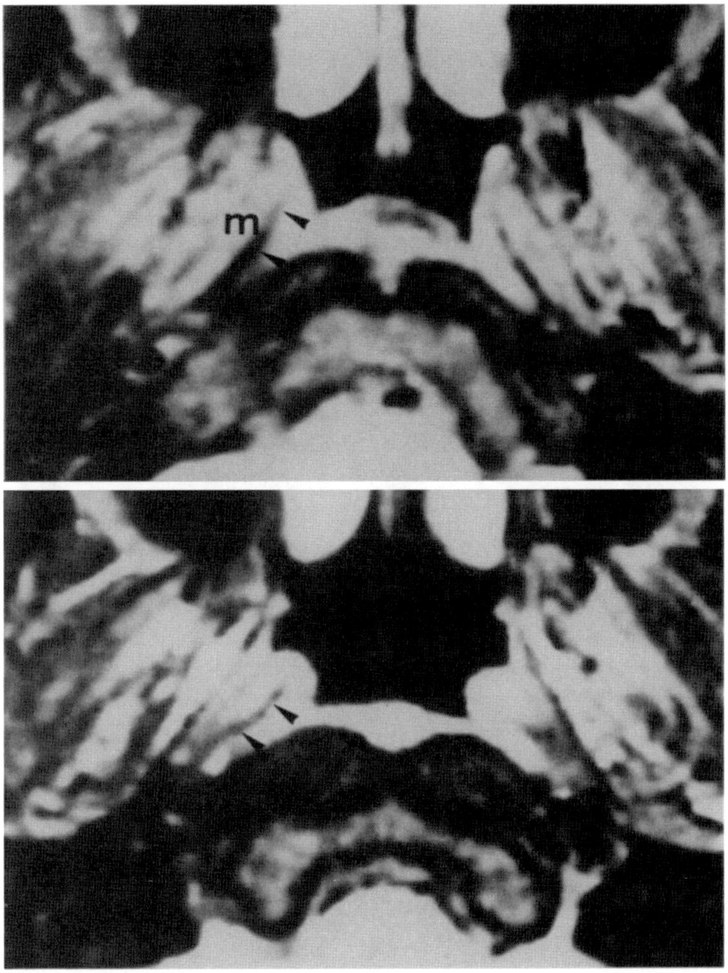

a

b

Fig. 7.16a, b. MRI of **a** upper and **b** lower halves of eustachian tube. Mucosa (*m*) and cartilage (*arrowheads*) of tube are clearly identified

muscle of both sides fused in the middle of the soft palate (Fig. 7.17b) in the section below Fig. 7.17a.

Based on these normal MRI findings around the eustachian tube, ten patients with NPC were evaluated by MRI before irradiation therapy. CT scan and tests for eustachian tube function were also carried out.

7.5.1 Comparison Between CT and MRI

The contrast between the tumor and soft tissue such as muscle was considerably greater with MRI than with CT, allowing clear identification of the tumor margin, especially when the tumor extended laterally or posteriorly and invaded

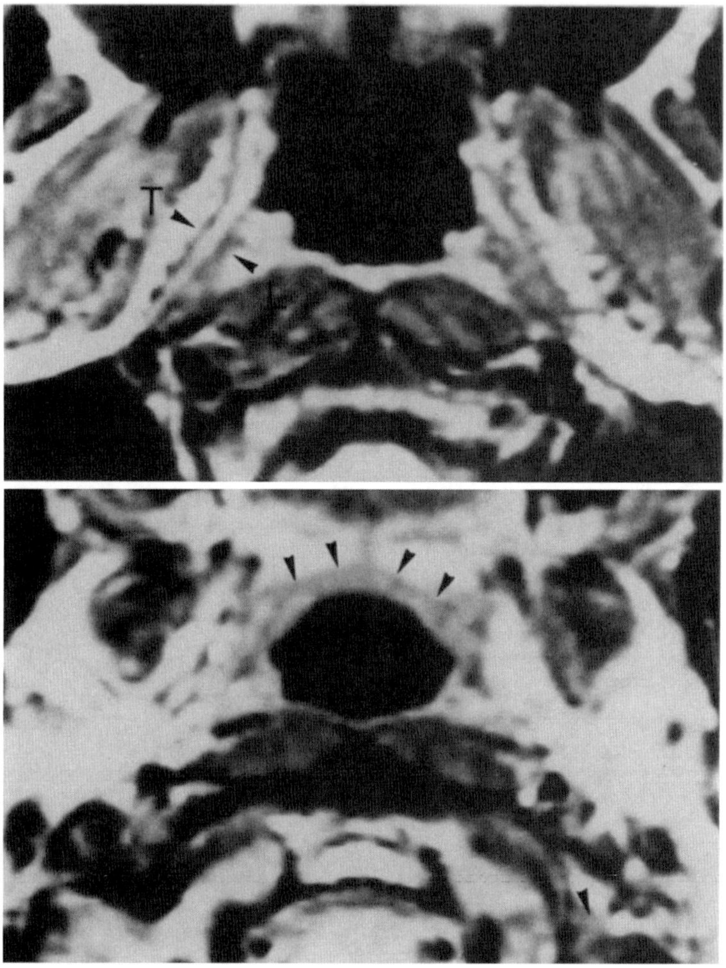

a

b

Fig. 7.17a, b. MRI below eustachian tube. **a** Tensor (*T*) and levator (*L*) muscles are identified. **b** Levator muscles of both sides fuse in middle of soft palate (*arrowheads*)

the pterygoid muscles and longus capitis muscle (patients 1, 4, 5, 8, 9, and 10; Fig. 7.18).

Lateral progression of the tumor can be evaluated by CT to some extent according to the change in the low-density areas representing fat in the parapharyngeal space. However, whether these changes were due to lateral displacement of normal tissue or invasion of the tumor itself was difficult to assess. Also, identification of fine structures in and around the eustachian tube was difficult by CT. On the other hand, as was shown in the controls, components of soft tissue including the tubal cartilage could be clearly distinguished by MRI. This allowed determination of the relation between the tumor and eustachian tube as well as the direction of tumor extension.

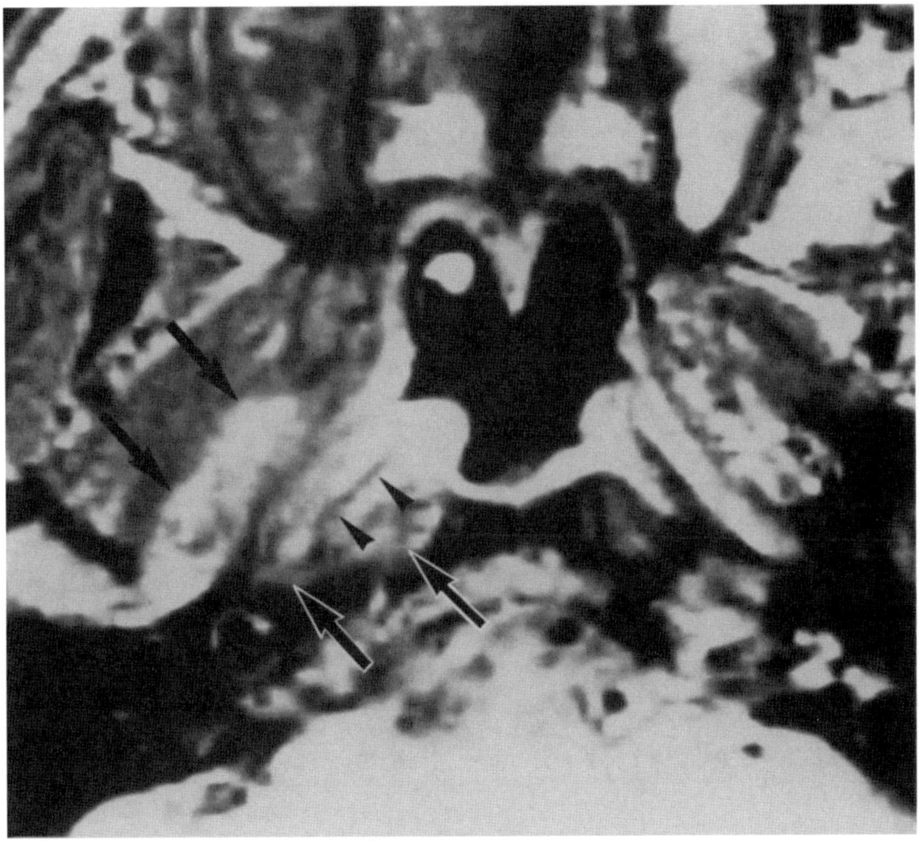

Fig. 7.18. MRI of patient 1. Tumor margin is clearly identified (*white arrows*) and the tubal cartilage (*arrowheads*) is not displaced

7.5.2 Invasion of Tumor to Eustachian Tube and Middle Ear Disease

OME and tubal functions in relation to MRI findings of the tube are summarized in Table 7.2. Otitis media was absent only in patients 1 and 2. In MRI of patient 1, the tumor filled the parapharyngeal space and extended to the area below the eustachian tube, but no displacement of the tubal cartilage was observed (Fig. 7.18). In patient 2, the tumor was located in the posterosuperior wall of the nasopharynx, and no abnormalities in the cartilage or the mucosa of the eustachian tube were noted (Fig. 7.19).

Unilateral OME and involvement of the tube by the tumor were noted in all the remaining patients by MRI. In patients 3, 4, 5, and 7, in whom a medium-sized tumor extended from Rosenmüller's fossa, the tubal cartilage was displaced laterally (Fig. 7.20). In patient 6, the tubal cartilage was in the normal position, but invasion of the tumor in the tube between the tubal cartilage and the tensor muscle was noted (Fig. 7.21). In patients 8 and 9, the tubal cartilage

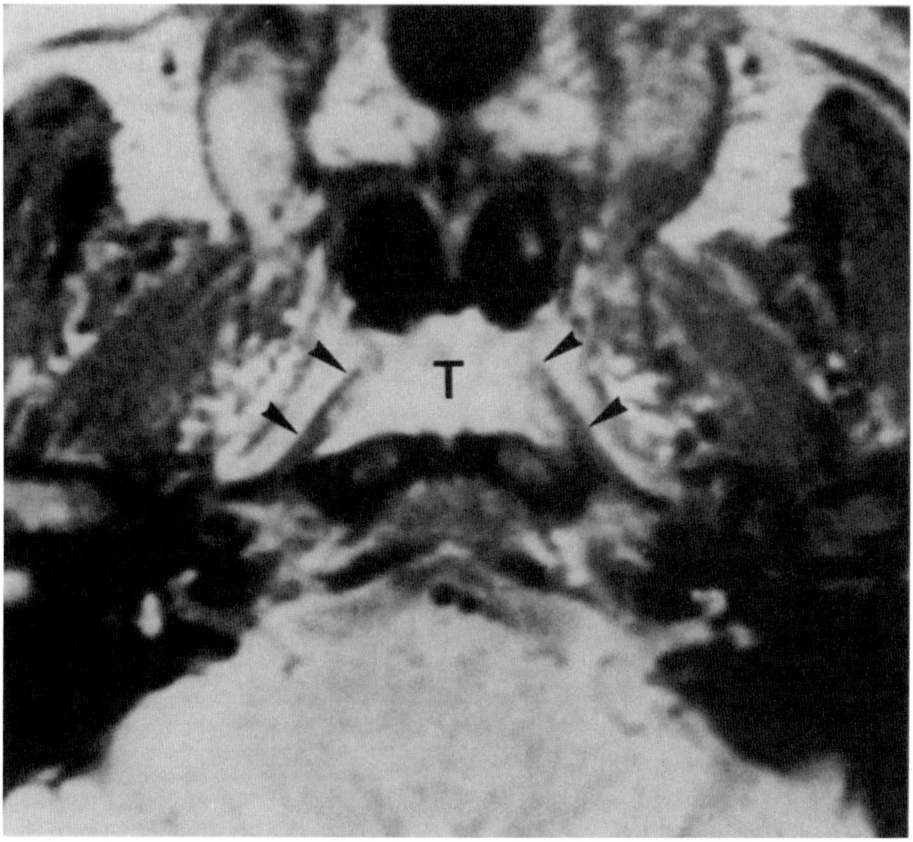

Fig. 7.19. MRI of patient 2. Tumor (*T*) is located in posterosuperior wall of nasopharynx. No displacement was found in tubal cartilage (*arrowheads*)

and muscles around the eustachian tube could not be identified because they were incorporated in a widely extended tumor.

Morphological abnormalities of the eustachian tube were consistently observed with MRI in all patients with NPC who developed OME. As was expected, OME was present when the tumor had widely extended around the eustachian tube. Interestingly, however, OME was also present in patients with moderately progressed tumors. In these patients, the primary lesion was located on the pharyngeal side of the eustachian tube, and no abnormalities were noted around the tubal isthmus. This indicates the importance of the spacial relationship between the tumor and the pharyngeal portion of the eustachian tube in the development of OME.

In patients 2 and 3, the tumors were of a similar size and located in the posterior wall, partially extending to Rosenmüller's fossa. However, patient 3 showed lateral displacement of the tubal cartilage and had OME (Fig. 7.20), while patient 2 exhibited neither displacement of the tubal cartilage nor ear dis-

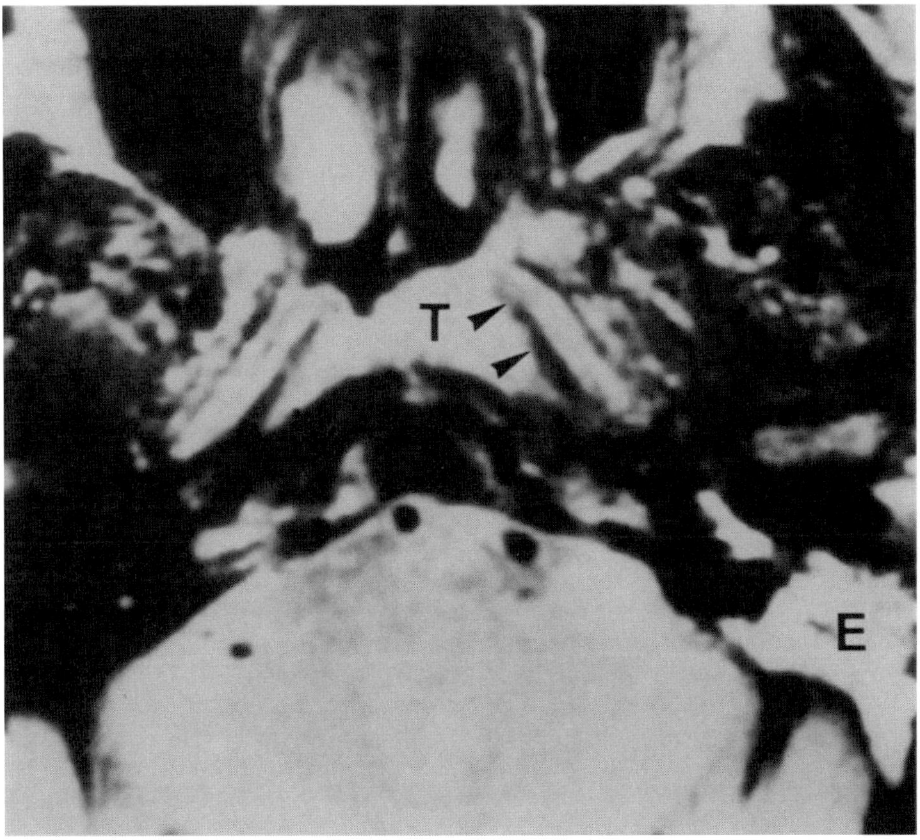

Fig. 7.20. MRI of patient 3. Tubal cartilage (*arrowheads*) is pushed outward by tumor (*T*). *E* middle ear effusion

ease (Fig. 7.19). These findings suggest that lateral displacement of the tubal cartilage by the tumor is an important factor in the development of OME. This view was also supported by the finding that OME was present in all four patients in whom lateral displacement of the tubal cartilage was noted. In contrast, OME was absent in patient 1, who had a large tumor located under the eustachian tube with no displacement of the tubal cartilage.

As for the relation between morphological changes in the eustachian tube and the function of the tube, the opening pressure was roughly proportionate to the size of the tumor around the tube, reflecting the extent of compression of the tube by the tumor (Table 7.2). The opening pressure was abnormally high only in patients 9 and 10, who exhibited marked invasion of the tumor around the tube, but the remaining patients showed normal or even lower opening pressure of the tube. Concerning the dynamic functions of the tube, the results of the positive pressure test were good in patients 4, 5, and 7, but the negative pressure test results were poor in all patients with OME, even in those whose eustachian

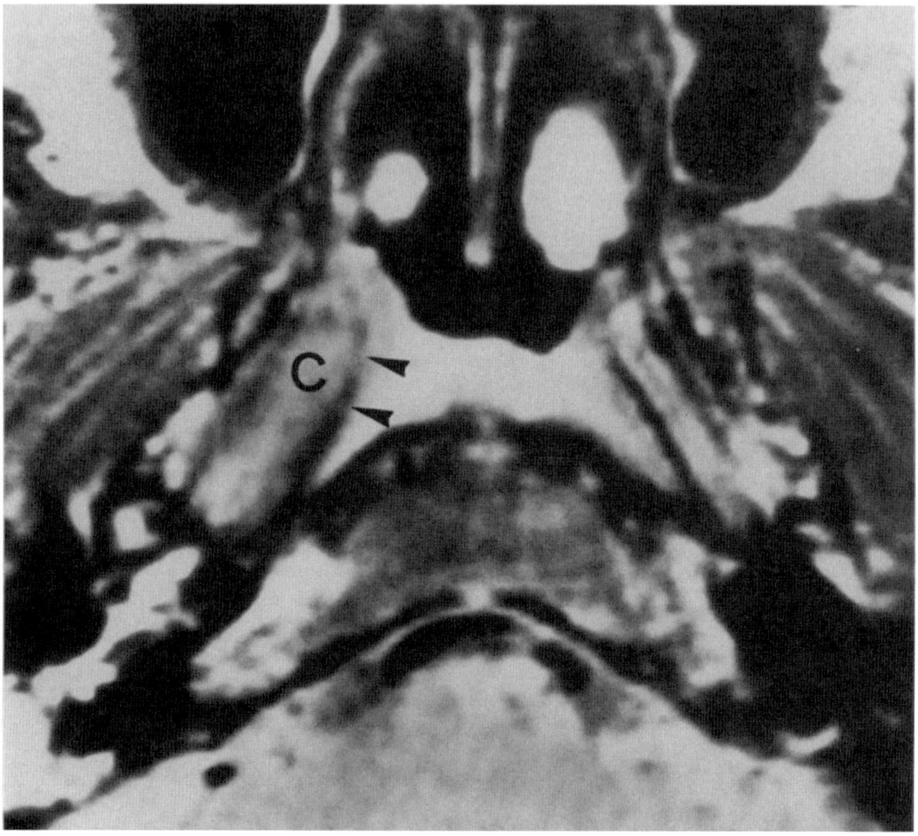

Fig. 7.21. MRI of patient 6. Carcinoma (*C*) invading tube is found between tubal cartilage (*arrowheads*) and tensor muscle

tube was considered to be normal by MRI. This suggested that impairment of relief of negative pressure is closely related to the development of OME.

By the lateral displacement of the tubal cartilage as observed even in the early stage of the tumor, contraction of the tensor muscle may not cause opening of the tubal lumen. This condition represents the tubal dysfunction in which negative middle ear pressure cannot be relieved by swallowing. The abnormal condition of the tube demonstrated both by MRI and the tubal function test appears to be responsible for production of OME in NPC patients.

7.5.3 Summary

MRI findings in ten patients with NPC in relation to the eustachian tube were as follows.

a) Compared with CT scan, MRI allowed more accurate evaluation of the extent of tumors that extend laterally or posteriorly from the Rosenmüller's fossa.

Table 7.1. MR findings and function of eustachian tube

Case	OME	MR findings	Tubal function		
			OP	PP	NP
1	–	No displacement of EC. Tumor is below ET			
2	–	No abnormal findings in EC, LVP, TVP			
3	+	EC is pushed outward	160	P	P
4	+	EC and LVP are pushed outward	190	G	P
5	+	EC is pushed outward and obscured	350	G	P
6	+	EC is obscured. Tumor invasion in ET	350	P	P
7	+	EC is pushed outward. Tumor invasion in ET	500	G	P
8	+	EC, LVP, TVP can not be identified	500	P	P
9	+	EC, LVP, TVP can not be identified	800	P	P
10	+	EC is pushed medially by the tumor in ET	640	P	P

OP opening pressure of the tube (mmH_2O), *PP* positive pressure test, *NP* negative pressure test, *G* good, *P* poor, *EC* eustachian tube cartilage, *LVP* levator muscle, *TVP* tensor muscle, *ET* eustachian tube

b) In NPC patients with OME, lateral displacement of the tubal cartilage, which impaired the ability to relieve negative middle ear pressure, was consistently observed.

7.6 Summary of Chapter

Contrary to our expectation, NPC was found to cause little stenosis or obstruction of the eustachian tube, as in the case of adenoids occupying the nasopharyngeal space. A large mass in the nasopharynx had little effect on the patency of the tube, indicating that simple obstruction of eustachian tube was unlikely to be the cause of OME. However, the degree of impairment of dynamic function of the tube, especially equalization of negative middle ear pressure by swallowing, was greatest in the early stage of the nasopharyngeal tumor, as was observed in the convalescent stage of OME. Ciliary clearance function of the tube was also significantly impaired in correlation with the degree of NPC, indicating some effect of inflammatory factors from the tumor on the eustachian tube. Involvement of inflammation in the development of OME in NPC was also suggested by a high PGE_2 level in the middle ear effusion in patients with NPC. Both impairment of dynamic function of the tube and inflammation were thought to be responsible for the development of OME even in NPC patients. Lateral displacement of the tubal cartilage by the tumor, which was demonstrated consistently by MRI, was found to be the condition that impaired the dynamic function of the tube, leading to the development of OME.

Although carcinoma of the nasopharynx is not a common disease except in limited areas of Asia, otolaryngologists should consider this disease when the patient complains of persistent OME, because ear symptoms are the only manifestation of this disease in about one-third of the patients.

References

Dickson RI (1981) Nasopharyngeal carcinoma: An evaluation of 209 patients. Laryngoscope 91:333–354

Druss JG (1940) Carcinoma of the nasopharynx with extension to the petrous pyramid. Report of case. Laryngoscope 50:359–365

Godtfredsen E, Lederman M (1965) Diagnostic and prognostic roles of ophthalmoneurologic signs and symptoms in malignant nasopharyngeal tumors. Am J Ophthalmol 59: 1063–1069

Panje WR (1981) Regression of head and neck carcinoma with a prostaglandin-synthesis inhibitor. Arch Otolaryngol 107:658–663

Sawaki S (1979) Basic and clinical study of nasopharyngeal carcinoma. J Otolaryngol Jap 82:1345–1351 (in Japanese)

Teoh TB (1957) Epidermoid carcinoma of the nasopharynx among Chinese: A study of 31 necropsies. J Path Bact 73:451–465

Thomas JA, Illescu V, Crowford DH, Ellouz R, Cammoun M, De-The G (1984) Expression of HLADR antigens in nasopharyngeal carcinoma: An immunohistological analysis of the tumour cells and infiltrating lymphocytes. Int J Cancer 33:813–819

Chapter 8
Middle Ear Disease and Eustachian Tube in Patients with Cleft Palate

Patients with cleft palate frequently suffer from middle ear disease such as OME. The cause of the high incidence of ear disease has not been determined, though several factors have been suggested as being involved in the etiology. Among them, velopharyngeal insufficiency, which causes contamination of the pharyngeal orifice of the eustachian tube by food or saliva, or nasal disease, such as paranasal sinusitis associated with cleft palate (Sataloff et al. 1952), have been thought to be responsible for middle ear disease. Some investigators have suggested that an abnormal course or insertion of palatal muscles (the levator and the tensor veli palatini muscles) causes dysfunction of the tube (Kriens 1975; Dickson 1976). Also, congenital anomaly of the eustachian tube including the tubal cartilage cannot be excluded.

Since the eustachian tube in patients with cleft palate is different in many ways from that of normal cases, this pathological condition is considered to provide important clues for the role of eustachian tube disorders in the development of OME in general.

Questions to be examined in the present study are: (a) Why is cleft palate frequently accompanied by ear disease? (b) what are the characteristics of eustachian tube dysfunction in cleft palate patient? and (c) what are the similarities or differences in OME between patients with and without cleft palate?

Eustachian tube function was examined by various tests, including endoscopy of the pharyngeal orifice of the tube and MRI as well as conventional tests.

8.1 Middle Ear Disease in Patients with Cleft Palate

Bluestone (1971) reported a high incidence of OME in patients with cleft palate. In the present study, the incidence of various middle ear diseases, including OME, was examined in cleft palate patient. The relation between ear disease and the type of cleft or its laterality were also examined to obtain basic data in the analysis of the role of eustachian tube dysfunction in the development of middle ear disease.

This study included 250 patients (500 ears) of all ages with cleft palate who visited our department with complaints of speech disturbance and disease in the ear or nose. Among them, 233 patients (466 ears) had undergone palatoplasty,

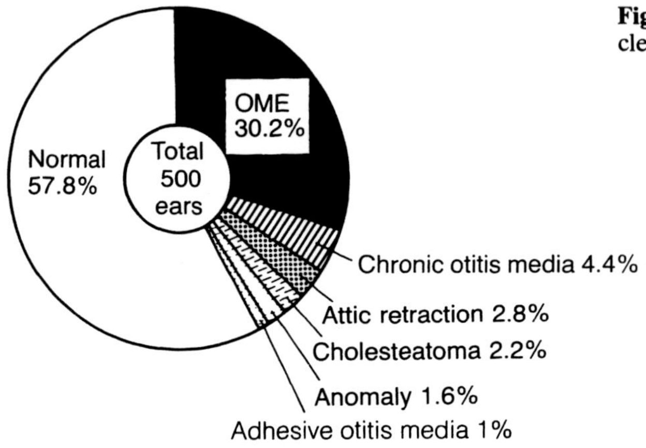

Fig. 8.1. Middle ear disease in cleft palate patients (500 ears)

and 17 (34 ears) had not been operated upon. To study the influence of velopharyngeal insufficiency upon middle ear disease, 16 patients (32 ears) with congenital velopharyngeal insufficiency without a cleft palate were also examined.

After inspection of the eardrum with a pneumatic otoscope, pure-tone audiometry and tympanometry were carried out in all patients. When OME was suspected, it was confirmed by myringotomy.

8.1.1 Frequency of Middle Ear Disease in Patients with Cleft Palate

The incidence of ear disease in patients with cleft palate was 42.2% of the 500 ears examined. Among them, OME was the most frequent disease, being observed in 30.2% of all ears tested; it represented 71.7% of middle ear diseases of the present subjects (Fig. 8.1). Other ear diseases were chronic otitis media, retraction pocket, cholesteatoma, and adhesive otitis media. However, acute otitis media was not observed in any of these patients.

Thus, cleft palate was associated with a high incidence of OME, suggesting a close relation between OME and dysfunction of the eustachian tube. Cleft palate patients should be followed up with respect to their ear disease as well as their speech problem.

8.1.2 Is Middle Ear Disease Related to Type or Laterality of Cleft?

As the severity of the cleft palate ranges from soft palate cleft to complete bilateral cleft, there may be an association between the type or laterality of cleft and the frequency of middle ear disease. Although Mitoma (1986) found no association here, this relation was reexamined in a large number of patients.

As shown in Fig. 8.2, no significant differences were noted in the incidence of middle ear disease among the various types of cleft, though the incidence was markedly low in patients with submucous cleft palate. Thus, the present results are in good agreement with those of earlier reports.

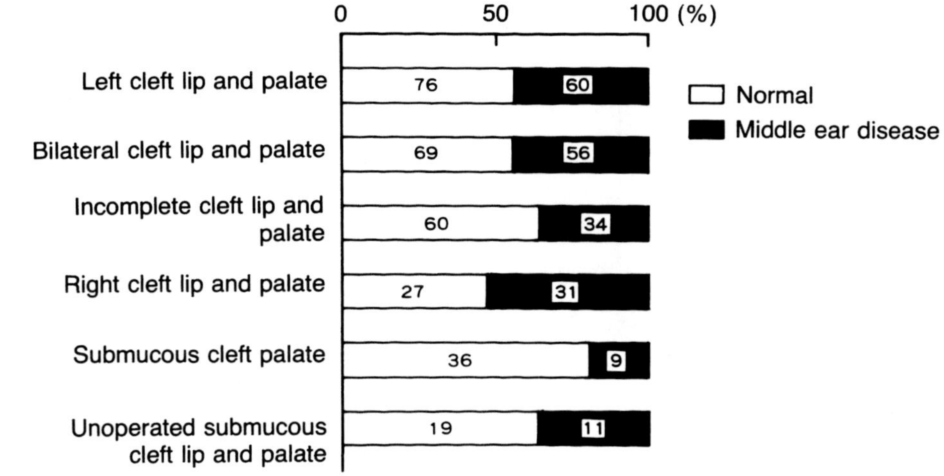

Fig. 8.2. Types of cleft and middle ear diseases

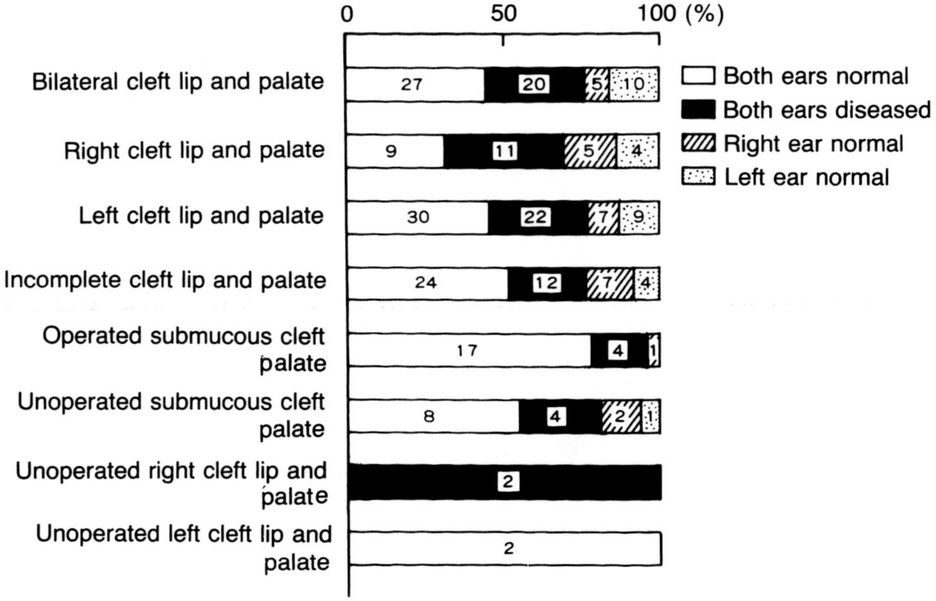

Fig. 8.3. Side of cleft and middle ear disease

The relation between the laterality of the cleft and middle ear disease was also examined. The patients were divided into four groups according to the condition of the ears because left-sided cleft is known to be more frequent than right-sided cleft: (a) patients whose ears were bilaterally normal; (b) those whose ears were bilaterally affected; (c) those whose left ear was affected; and (d) those whose right ear was affected. As shown in Fig. 8.3, regardless of the type of cleft, more

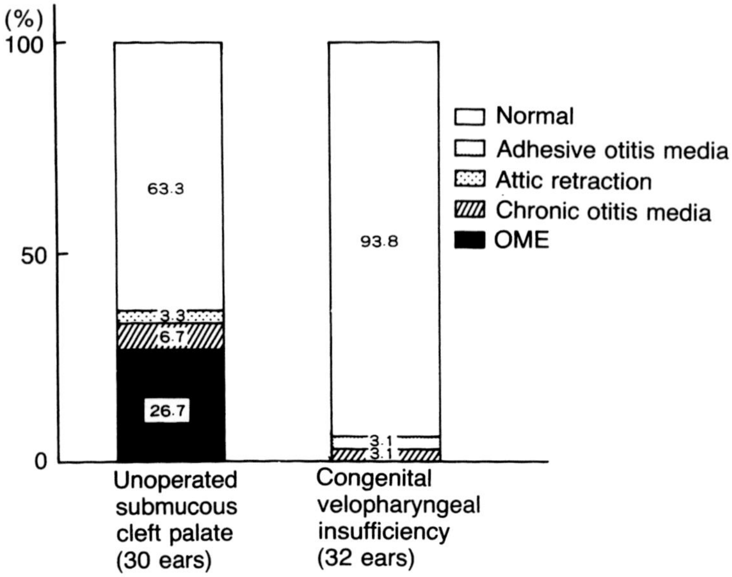

Fig. 8.4. Velopharyngeal insufficiency and middle ear disease

than 77.7% of the patients showed the same condition in both ears, namely either bilaterally affected or bilaterally normal. In addition, the frequency of middle ear disease in unilateral cleft was not significantly high on the cleft side. Thus, there was no correlation between laterality of the cleft and ear disease.

These results suggest that bilateral eustachian tubes have the same anatomical condition in middle ear disease, regardless of the type or laterality of cleft.

8.1.3 Velopharyngeal Insufficiency and Middle Ear Disease

Spriestersbach et al. (1962), Paulsen (1964), and Okazaki et al. (1980) suggested a relation between velopharyngeal insufficiency and middle ear disease. In this section, this relation is again examined in selected cases, i.e., congenital velopharyngeal insufficiency (CVPI) and submucous cleft palate (SCP). Though both groups have velopharyngeal insufficiency, SCP patients exhibit abnormality in the course and attachment of palatal muscles. The incidence of middle ear disease in 30 ears of unoperated SCP patients and 32 ears of CVPI patients was compared.

As shown in Fig. 8.4, the incidence of middle ear disease was 37% of the SCP group, while the CVPI group had a significantly lower incidence of ear disease (6.2%). None of the CVPI patients had OME, despite notable insufficiency of velopharyngeal closure. Thus, there was no correlation between OME and velopharyngeal insufficiency.

Contamination of the nasopharynx from the oral cavity due to incomplete closure of the velopharynx has been considered to be one of the causes of middle ear disease in cleft palate patients. However, the incidence of middle ear disease in CVPI patients was significantly lower than SMCP patients who had abnormality in the palatal muscles in addition to the velopharyngeal insufficiency. These findings suggest that incomplete closure of the nasopharynx is not a primary factor in the pathogenesis of middle ear disease in cleft palate patients.

8.1.4 Summary

The results of 500 ears of cleft palate patients were generally consistent with those of earlier reports.

a) About half of the ears showed middle ear disease, including OME, which requires otological treatment.
b) There was no difference in the incidence of middle ear disease in relation to the type or laterality of the cleft, suggesting equal involvement of a pathological condition in both eustachian tubes.
c) Contamination from the oral cavity due to velopharyngeal insufficiency is unlikely to be the cause of middle ear disease.

8.2 Pharyngeal Orifice of Eustachian Tube in Cleft Palate

Abnormalities of the course and attachment of the palatal muscles (tensor and levator veli palatini muscles) in cleft palate patients have been well documented. Since these muscles are also closely related to the eustachian tube, the movement of the tube during swallowing and phonation may be different in patients without clefts. By endoscopic observation of cleft palate patients, Mitoma et al. (1985) reported contradictory motions of the pharyngeal orifice of the tube during these activities. Although endoscopic findings of the pharyngeal orifice do not always allow evaluation of the entire tube, abnormalities around the orifice indicate tubal dysfunction, even when the upper portions of the tube, such as the isthmus, are normal.

In the present study, movement of the pharyngeal orifice of the tube was examined during swallowing, phonation, and opening of the mouth as in yawning, by a flexible endoscope (Type-P, Olympus) through the nose.

8.2.1 Middle Ear Disease and Abnormal Movement of Pharyngeal Orifice

As shown in Fig. 8.5, the pharyngeal orifice of the tube opened, closed, or closure remained unchanged during swallowing, phonation, or opening of the mouth. The pharyngeal orifice opened in 58.5% of cleft palate patients during swallowing, and it opened in 25.8% during opening of the mouth. Thus, the ability to open the pharyngeal orifice was found to be impaired in cleft palate patients.

The ears in which the pharyngeal orifice of the tube did not open could be divided into two groups. In one group, the orifice was not funnel-shaped and the tensor muscle could be identified during swallowing; the other group showed no opening of the orifice due to insufficient contraction of the tensor muscle. In

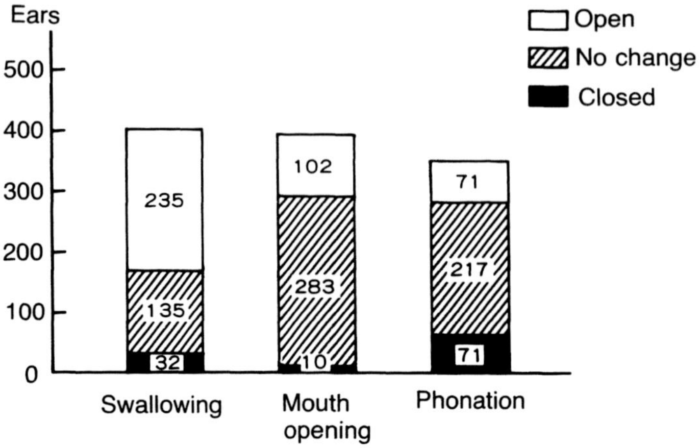

Fig. 8.5. Movement of tubal orifice in swallowing, phonation, and mouth opening

some cases, the pharyngeal orifice was closed either by the levator muscle (Fig. 8.6), which forms the floor of the eustachian tube, or by displacement of the posterior lip of the tube over the orifice.

To examine the relation between the abnormal motion of the orifice and disease in the middle ear, the frequency of ear disease was compared between ears that showed tubal opening during swallowing, phonation, or opening of the mouth and those that showed no opening of the orifice during these actions. As shown in Fig. 8.7, middle ear disease was found in only 23% of ears where the pharyngeal orifice of the tube opened. In this group, OME, chronic otitis media, retraction pocket, and cholesteatoma occurred with nearly the same frequency. In contrast, in the ears that showed no opening of the orifice, the incidence of middle ear disease was 62%. Among these middle ear diseases, OME comprised 91%.

These abnormal motions of the pharyngeal orifice can be ascribed to the anomalous course or attachment of the levator muscle (Kriens 1975) (Fig. 8.8) or congenital hypoplasia of the tensor muscle (Fara et al. 1970). Opening failure of the eustachian tube due to such abnormality appeared to be responsible for the high incidence of OME in cleft palate patients.

8.2.2 Relation Between Abnormalities of Pharyngeal Orifice and Eustachian Tube Function

As the opening failure of the tube was closely related to OME, the function of the eustachian tube was examined in 137 ears of cleft palate patients who underwent endoscopic examination. Among them, 35 ears showed opening of the pharyngeal orifice, while 102 ears showed no opening.

Ventilatory function of the tube was examined with respect to the opening pressure of the tube at rest and the dynamic function of the tube during swallowing. When a pressure of +200 mmH_2O could not be applied due to incomplete

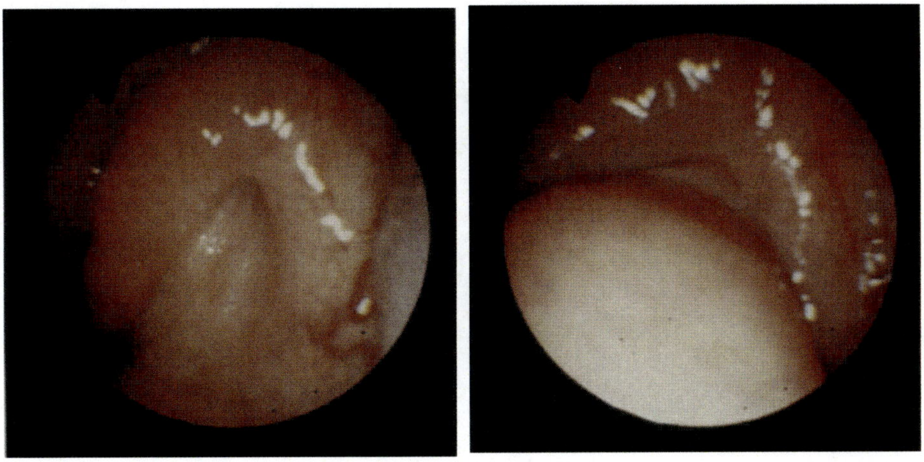

Fig. 8.6. Abnormal movement of pharyngeal orifice of eustachian tube. Levator veli palatini muscle closes orifice during swallowing

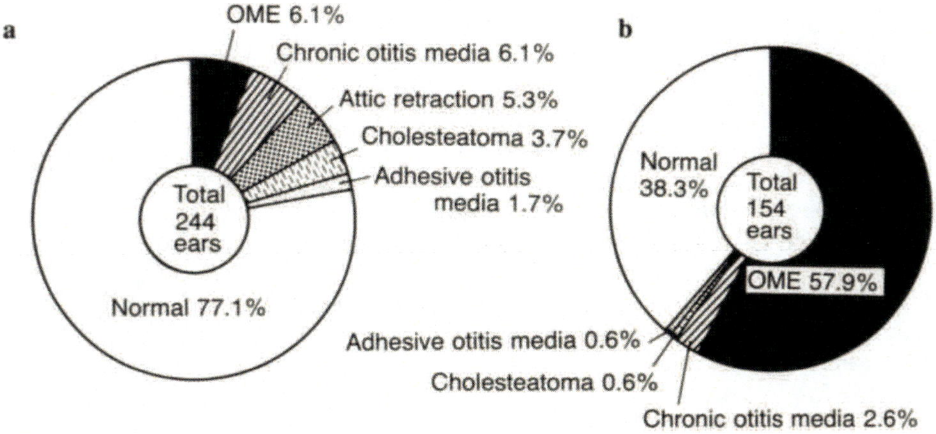

Fig. 8.7a, b. Incidence of middle ear disease. **a** Patients whose tubal orifices open during swallowing. **b** Patients whose tubal orifices do not open

closure of the tube, the pressure was reduced to 150, 100, or 50 mmH_2O. The clearance function of the tube was examined by a dye test.

In the ears in which the pharyngeal orifice opened during swallowing, the results of the positive pressure test were good in 54.0%, and those of the negative pressure test were also good in 45% (Fig. 8.9). On the other hand, in the ears that showed no opening of the pharyngeal orifice, the results of the positive pressure test were good in 55.0% of ears, which was comparable with that in the group with tubal opening. However, the ability to equalize negative pressure by

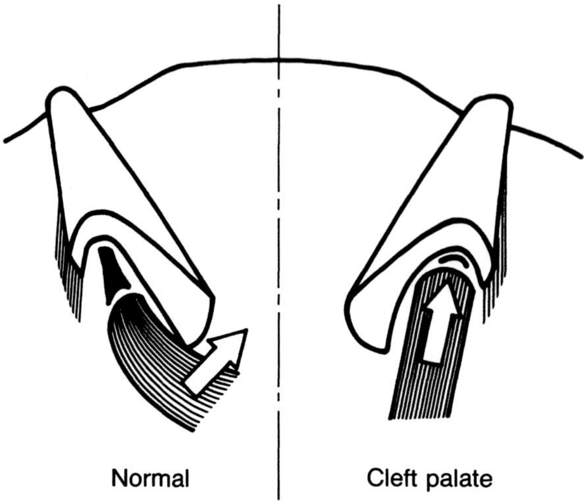

Fig. 8.8. Closure of pharyngeal orifice of eustachian tube by levator muscle

swallowing was extremely poor (93%) in this group. Both groups showed good clearance function of the tube. Thus, marked impairment of tubal function to equalize negative middle ear pressure in the ears in which the orifice did not open, was demonstrated.

Though the results of the negative pressure test in the first group were not satisfactory in more than half of the patients, 88.9% of the ears without middle ear effusion in this first group showed good results in the test. Certainly, in the second group in which the orifice did not open, the results of the negative pressure test were poor in 83%, despite no effusion in the ear.

These results suggest that the dynamic function of the tube is significantly impaired in the ears which have no tubal opening at the pharyngeal orifice. Although endoscopic observation is limited to the pharyngeal part of the tube, disturbance of the tubal orifice is considered to be closely related to the development of OME.

8.2.3 Summary

The relation between endoscopic findings of the pharyngeal orifice of the tube in cleft palate patients and eustachian tube function or middle ear disease are as follows.

a) Abnormal movement of the pharyngeal orifice of the tube was frequently observed during swallowing or other actions. The incidence of middle ear disease including OME was significantly high in the ears in which the orifice of the tube did not open.
b) In the ears in which the pharyngeal orifice did not open, relief of negative middle ear pressure during swallowing was markedly impaired, suggesting that the impaired dynamic function of the tube in cleft palate is related to the development of OME.

Fig. 8.9. Movement of tubal orifice and its function

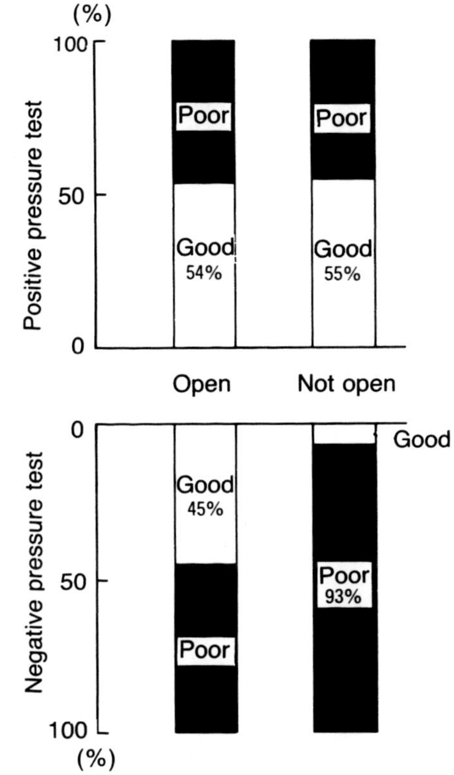

8.3 Eustachian Tube Function in OME Patients with Cleft Palate

To clarify the pathogenetic factors of OME in cleft palate patients, eustachian tube function was examined in 100 ears of patients with OME (4–50 years old). In addition to testing the ventilatory function and clearance function of the tube, manosonometry, which examines the closing failure of the eustachian tube, was performed. As the closure of the tube at rest was found to be inadequate in cleft palate patients, the sniffing test was also carried out to examine whether nasopharyngeal pressure is transmitted to the middle ear.

8.3.1 Ventilatory and Clearance Functions of Eustachian Tube in Cleft Palate

In OME patients with a cleft palate, the minimum pressure for tubal opening at rest was 276 mmH_2O, which was significantly lower than that in the normal ear (354 mmH_2O; Fig. 8.10). The median value of opening pressure of the tube in cleft palate patients was also lower than normal.

Opening pressure of the tube reflects the patency of the tube or its ability to close at rest. Surina and Jagr (1969) observed reductions in the elasticity of the structures in and around the tube in cleft palate patients. The low opening pressure which characterizes the eustachian tube of cleft palate patients may be

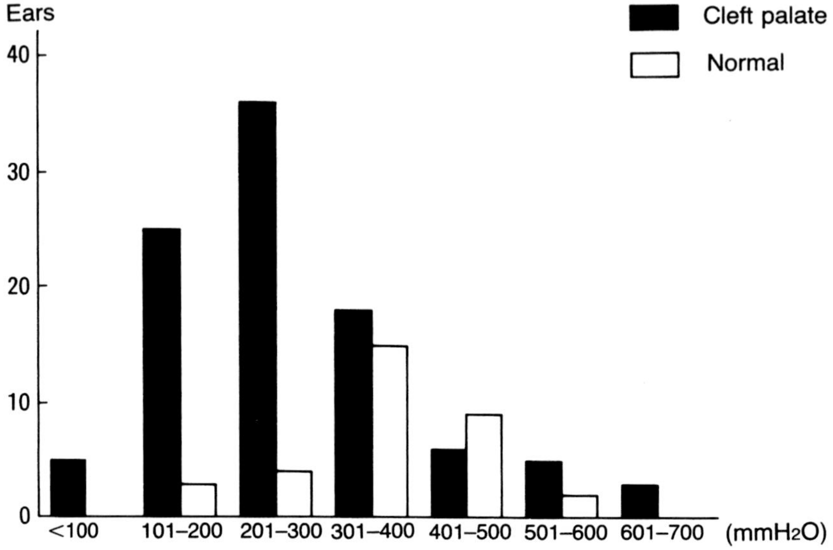

Fig. 8.10. Opening pressure of tube in cleft palate patients with OME

derived from this anatomical abnormality.

With regard to the dynamic function of the tube in OME patients with cleft palate, the relief of positive pressure was good in 50 ears (50%), but relief of negative pressure was extremly poor in 93.0% (Fig. 8.11). As demonstrated in Chap. 5 on non-cleft patients, impairment of dynamic function of the tube in OME, especially poor relief of negative middle ear pressure, was considered to be a common pathogenic condition of the eustachian tube regardless of cleft palate.

Incomplete closure of the eustachian tube was detected by manosonometry. Among 43 ears with OME, incomplete closure was noted in 53.5% (23 ears), indicating a marked reduction in the closing force of the tube in cleft palate patients. On the other hand, closing failure of the tube was noted in 24% of the 96 ears of OME patients without a cleft palate (Fig. 8.12).

These results indicate that the eustachian tube in cleft palate patients is characterized by a weak tubal closing force and the inability of the tube to relieve negative middle ear pressure. These findings are similar to those observed in the floppy tube reported by Bluestone (1971) and in closing failure of the tube reported by Falk et al. (1984).

The sniffing test was performed in 56 ears with OME. By sniffing, negative middle ear pressure developed in only 19.6% (11 ears), which is comparable with OME patients without cleft palate. As the opening pressure was extremely low (mean 97.3 ± 95.5 mmH_2O) in these patients, negative pressure may develop in the middle ear cavity by sniffing (Fig. 8.13). Since negative middle ear pressure could not be relieved by swallowing in these patients, it is suggested that sniffing may produce negative pressure in the middle ear cavity in a certain number of cleft palate patient.

Fig. 8.11. Dynamic ventilatory function of tube in cleft palate patients with OME

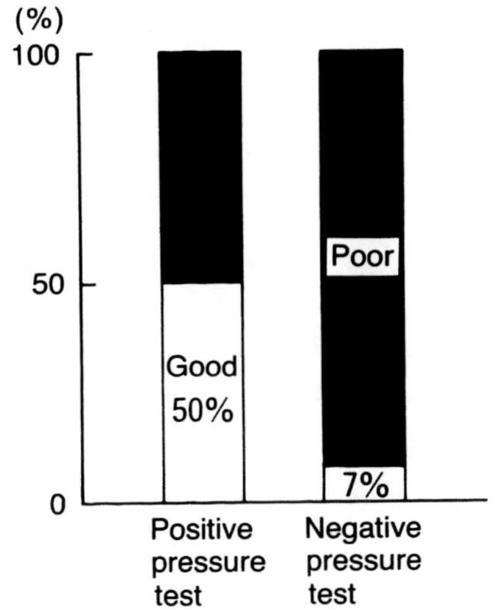

Fig. 8.12. Incidence of closing failure of tube in cleft palate patients with OME

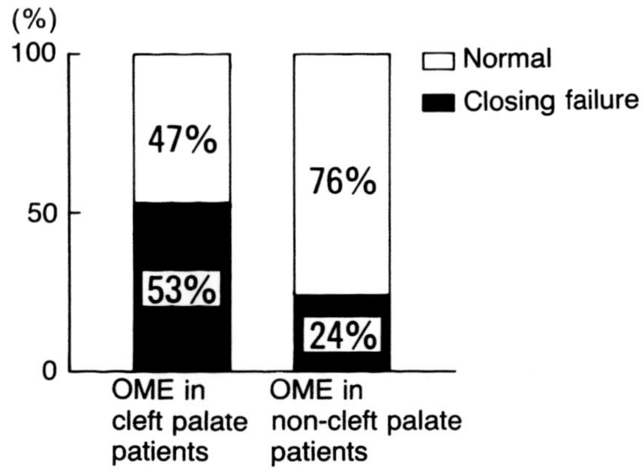

Clearance function of the tube was normal in 72.7% (48 ears) of these patients (Fig. 8.14) in constrast to marked impairment in 60%–70% of OME patients without cleft palate. Therefore, inflammatory factors impairing ciliary activity of the tube may not be important in the pathogenesis of OME in cleft palate.

8.3.2 Summary

Examination of eustachian tube function in 100 cleft palate patients with OME revealed the following.

a) The opening pressure of the tube was lower than normal, suggesting that the tube in cleft palate is rather patent at rest. Closing failure of the tube was observed in more than 50% of the patients. A characteristic of

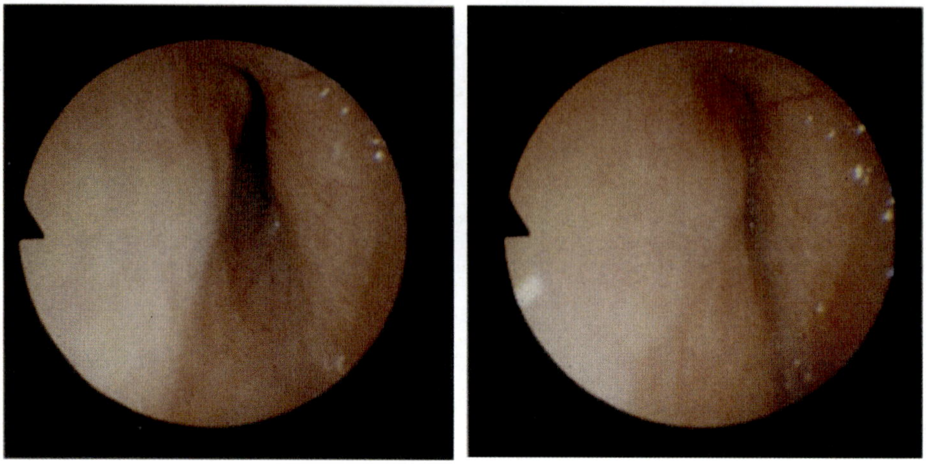

Fig. 8.13. Lock of pharyngeal orifice of tube during sniffing (right)

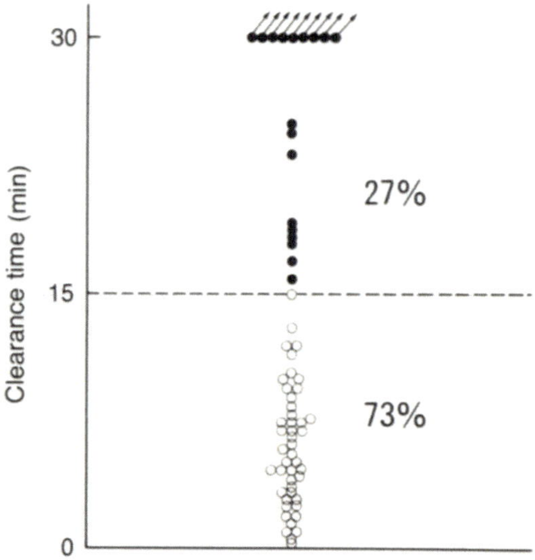

Fig. 8.14. Clearance function of tube in cleft palate patients with OME

the tubal dysfunction in cleft palate patients appears to be a failure to maintain the tubal lumen under normal conditions.

b) The results of the negative pressure test during swallowing were poor in most cases, as in OME patients without cleft palate.
c) Sniffing caused frequent negative middle ear pressure in the group which showed low opening pressure of the tube. However, this was seen in less than 20% of cleft palate patients, suggesting that this action has little influence on the development of OME.

8.4 Eustachian Tube Function in Unilateral, Convalescent, and Recurrent OME

The eustachian tube of cleft palate patients in different stages of OME was examined to clarify whether the characteristic findings of the ear in cleft palate obtained in the previous section were valid or not. In patients with unilateral OME, tubal function in the normal ear was examined and compared with that in the affected ear. Tubal function in recurrent OME and in the convalescent stage of OME was also examined. All tests were performed with consent of patients.

8.4.1 Eustachian Tube Function in Patients with Unilateral OME

The opening pressure of tubes in 16 patients (32 ears) with unilateral OME was examined. The mean opening pressure in the normal ears was 283 ± 166 mmH_2O, but it was significantly lower in ears with OME (197 ± 76 mmH_2O; Fig. 8.15). However, the opening pressure of the tube in normal ears was also lower than that in non-cleft controls. Thus, the eustachian tube in cleft palate patients appears to be patent even in the unaffected ear in unilateral OME.

Concerning the dynamic function of the tube, relief of positive pressure was good in 71% of the ears without OME, but it was good in only 47% of the ears with OME. The results of the negative pressure test were more definite than those of the positive pressure test. They were poor in 69% of ears without OME, but 88% of the ears with OME showed impaired relief of negative pressure (Fig. 8.16). Thus, both impairment of the dynamic function of the tube and weak closing force of the tube in cleft palate patients was again indicated by comparison of the ears with unilateral OME.

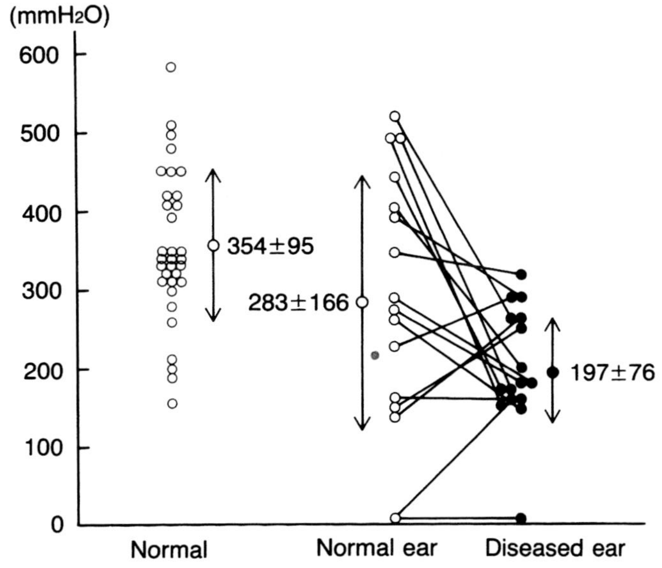

Fig. 8.15. Opening pressure of tube in affected ear of unilateral OME

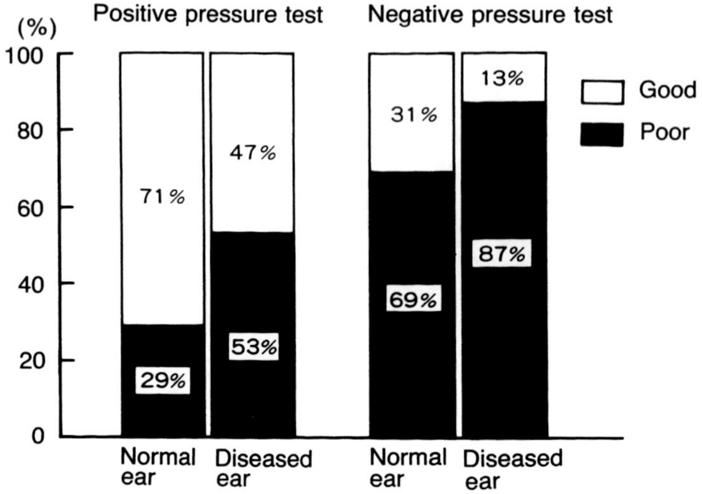

Fig. 8.16. Difference in dynamic ventilatory function of tube between affected and unaffected ears

8.4.2 Eustachian Tube Function in Convalescent Stage of OME in Cleft Palate

In the convalescent stage of OME, tubal function in 18 ears of cleft palate patients was examined. These patients showed no signs of OME by repeated inspection of the eardrum, audiometry, and tympanometry for more than 1 month after displacement of the tympanostomy tube.

The mean opening pressure of the tube was 341 ± 166 mmH_2O, which was comparable with that in the normal controls without cleft palate. The results of the positive pressure test were good in 78.0% (14 ears), but those of negative pressure test were poor in 83.3% (15 ears; Fig. 8.17).

The poor relief of the negative pressure in the convalescent stage of OME was similar to that in ears of cleft palate patients with OME. These results also indicate marked inability to relieve negative middle ear pressure in cleft palate patients. This may be a predisposing factor in these patients for the development of middle ear disease.

8.4.3 Eustachian Tube Function in Recurrent OME

This study included 31 ears that required over two insertions of a tympanostomy tube. The mean opening pressure of the tube was 221 ± 123 mmH_2O, which was significantly lower than the mean of 98 ears of all cleft palate patients with OME (278 ± 136 mmH_2O; Fig. 8.18). The results of the positive pressure test were good in 51.6% (16 ears), but those of the negative pressure test were poor in 94% (29 ears; Fig. 8.19).

The low opening pressure of the tube in patients with recurrent OME suggested that patency of the tube is a causative factor in the recurrence of OME. Impairment of the dynamic function of the tube was also seen in these patients.

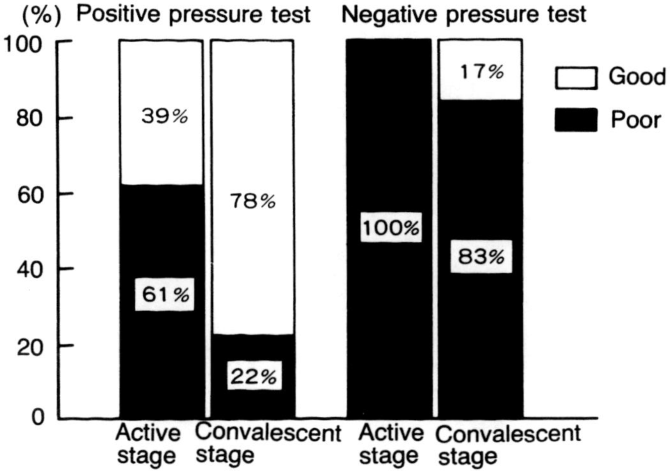

Fig. 8.17. Dynamic ventilatory function of tube in patients with OME in convalescent stage

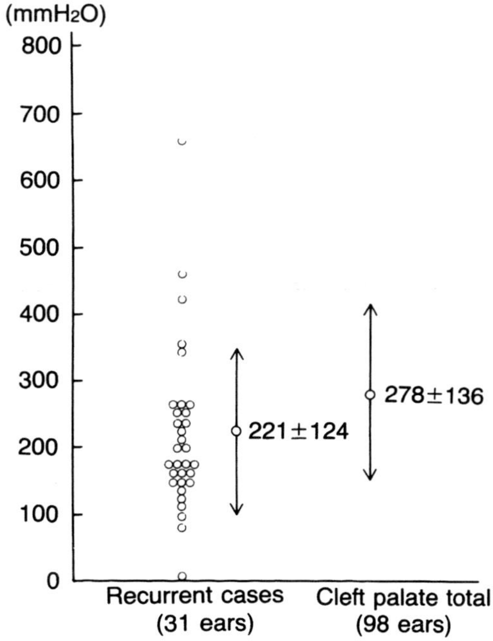

Fig. 8.18. Opening pressure of tube in patients with recurrent OME

In the patients with recurrent OME, the clearance function of the tube was normal in 87.5%, suggesting less impairment of ciliary activity of the tube. Thus, inflammation may play a minor role in the development of OME in cleft palate patients.

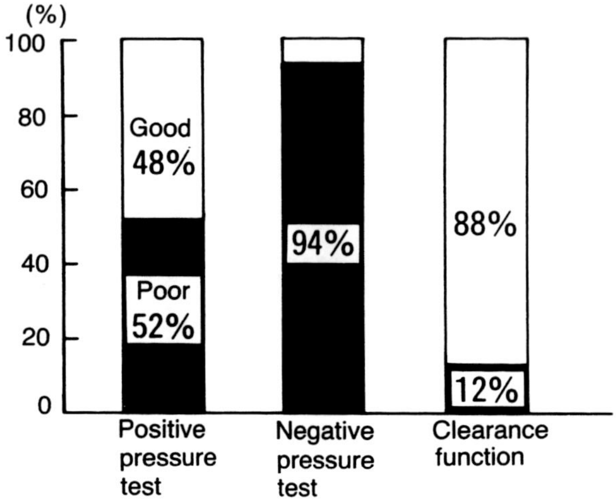

Fig. 8.19. Eustachian tube function in patients with recurrent OME

8.4.4 Summary

Eustachian tube function in cleft palate patients with unilateral, convalescent, and recurrent OME can be summarized as follows.

a) Opening pressure of the tube was low even in normal ears, and more than 50% of these ears were incapable of relieving negative middle ear pressure during swallowing.
b) The results of the negative pressure test were also poor in patients in the convalescent state of OME, suggesting that impairment of dynamic function of the tube is a predisposing factor for OME in cleft palate patients.
c) The opening pressure of the tube was significantly low in patients with recurrent OME as compared with all cleft palate patients with OME, indicating that patency of the tube was related to persistent OME. The clearance function of the tube, however, was almost normal. Thus, inflammatory factors were thought to be negligible in the development of OME in cleft palate.

8.5 MRI of Eustachian Tube in Cleft Palate

Morphological studies of the eustachian tube in cleft palate patients have been conducted mainly by anatomical study (Dickson 1976; Latham et al. 1980) and endoscopy of the pharyneal orifice of the tube (Mitoma et al. 1985). Radiographic examination of the eustachian tube and CT scan have also been employed. However, clear visualization of the tube with its surrounding structures was difficult even with these methods. As stated in the previous chapter on nasopharyngeal carcinoma, MRI was found to be useful for evaluation of the eustachian tube with its surrounding structures, such as tubal cartilage, mucosa, and muscles related to the tube.

8.5.1 MRI Findings in Cleft Palate

The tubal cartilage provides the framework for the eustachian tube; it helps the action of the tensor muscle in opening the tube. Malformation of the tubal cartilage, and abnormal courses of the tubal muscles in cleft palate patients were evaluated by MRI. The following are representative cases.

Case 1. This was a 50-year-old male with left complete cleft lip and palate (palate unoperated), who had right OME and left chronic otitis media. The tubal cartilage curved medially at the pharyngeal side, forming a cuplike contour (Fig. 8.20a). The high-signal area lateral to the cartilage represented the mucosal layer of the tube with mucous glands or mucus. The levator muscles were located laterally to their normal positions, without joining in the midline of the palate (Fig. 8.20b). In relation to the eustachian tube, these muscles were positioned higher than normal, almost on the same level as the lower part of the tubal cartilage.

Case 2. This was a 12-year-old male with submucous cleft, who had bilateral chronic otitis media. A similar cuplike curve at the distal part of the tubal cartilage was observed (Fig. 8.21a). The course of the levator muscles was also abnormal; they did not fuse in the midline but terminated in the posterior margin of the palatal bone (Fig. 8.21b).

Case 3. This was a 36-year-old male with right complete cleft lip and palate (palate unoperated) without middle ear disorder. Curvature of the tubal cartilage less than that in the above two cases was also observed in this patient (Fig. 8.22a). The levator muscles were positioned more laterally than normal and ran in the anterior direction without joining each other (Fig. 8.22b).

Among eight cleft palate patients examined by MRI, a cup-shaped tubal cartilage was noted in all cases, and the levator muscle was located lateral to the eustachian tube, running almost anteriorly.

Thick soft tissue, which represents the mucosal lining of the eustachian tube rich in secretory glands or mucus, was consistently observed lateral to the tubal cartilage. These pathological structures of the tubal cartilage and muscles and abnormalities of the tubal mucosa are considered to be responsible for the vulnerability of cleft palate patients to ear disease.

In the MRI of normal controls, the levator muscles ran below the tubal cartilage anteromedially, forming the so-called levator muscle sling (Fig. 7.17b). As shown in the present study, however, the levator of cleft palate patients ran anteriorly lateral to the tubal cartilage at a level higher than normal. Consequently, contraction of the levator in this abnormal course and position may result in invagination of the muscle into the tubal lumen between the tensor and the tubal cartilage. These processes are in close agreement with the endoscopic findings of contradictory movements, in which the pharyngeal orifice of the tube is obstructed by the levator contraction during swallowing or phonation.

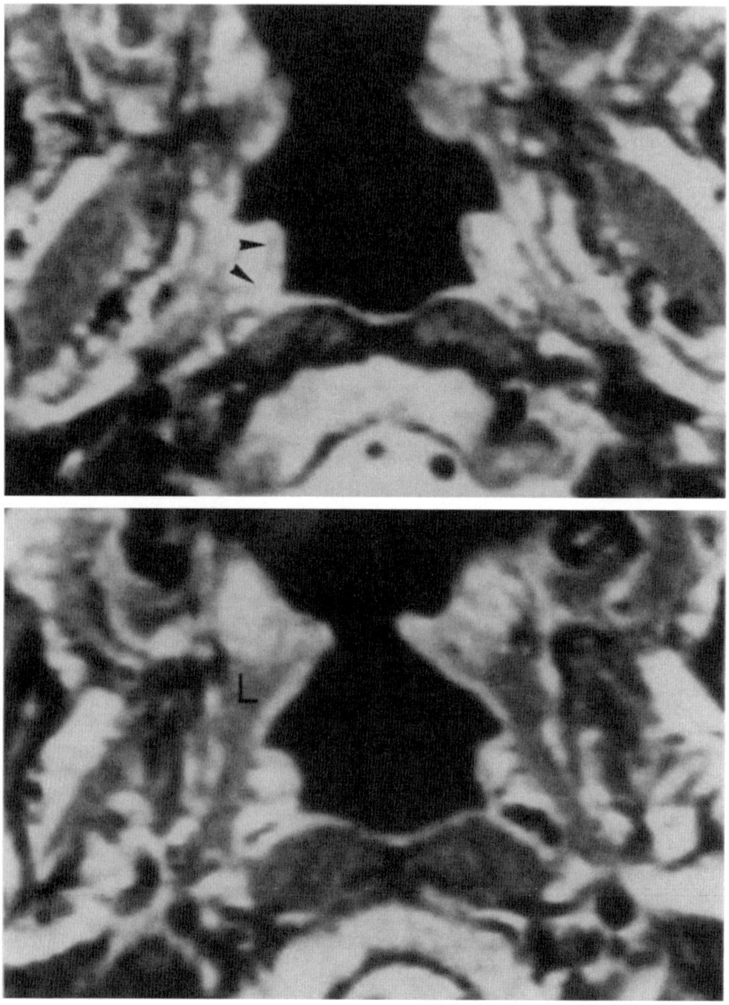

a

b

Fig. 8.20a, b. MRI of eustachian tube of patient 1. **a** Tubal cartilage is cup-shaped (arrowheads). **b** Levator muscle (*L*) is located lateral to its normal position

8.5.2 Summary

MRI findings of the eustachian tube in cleft palate patients can be summarized as follows.

a) Abnormal curvature of the tubal cartilage and thickening of the tubal mucosa were observed in the pharyngeal end of the tube.
b) Abnormal course and position of the levator muscle in relation to the eustachian tube was demonstrated by MRI.
c) Combined abnormalities of the tubal cartilage, muscles, and mucosa were considered to be responsible for eustachian tube dysfunction and the frequent occurrence of middle ear disease.

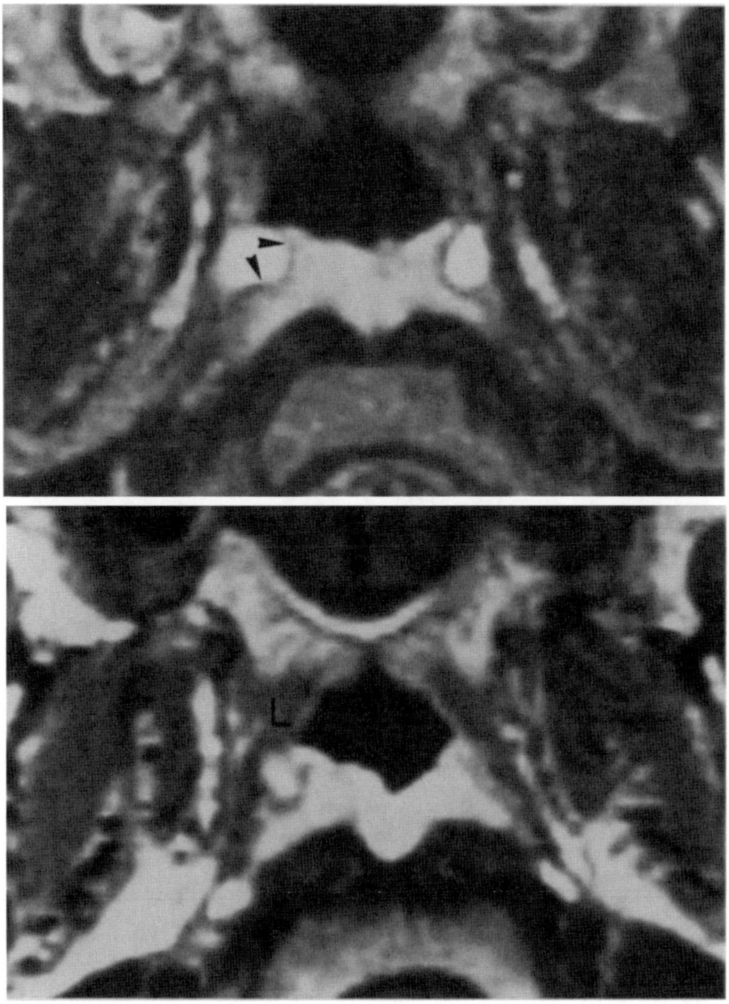

a
b

Fig. 8.21a, b. MRI of eustachian tube of patient 2. **a** Tubal cartilage is curved medially (arrowheads). **b** Levator muscle (*L*) is located lateral to its normal position

8.6 Summary of Chapter

Diseases of the middle ear, including OME, were found to occur frequently in patients with a cleft palate, and the importance of otological care for cleft palate patients was reemphasized.

Characteristic features of the eustachian tube in cleft palates were that the tube was generally patent and inadequately closed at rest, indicating it to be an inherent impairment of the tube. On the other hand, poor tubal opening, especially impairment of negative pressure equalization during swallowing, was demonstrated under several conditions of OME, such as in the unaffected ear in

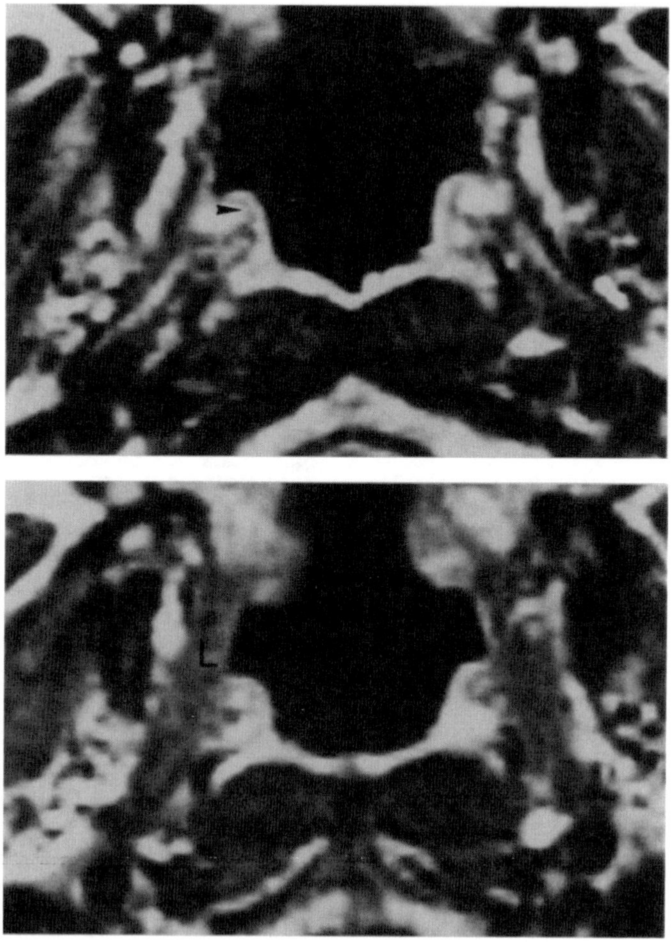

a

b

Fig. 8.22a, b. MRI of eustachian tube of patient 3. **a** Curve of tubal cartilage is not prominent (*arrowhead*). **b** Below **a** (4–5 mm), levator muscle (*L*) runs anteriorly

unilateral OME or ears in the convalescent stage of OME. From these results, along with MRI findings of curvature of the tubal cartilage and mucosal thickening, the framework and tubal lumen are considered to be loosely closed but not to open readily during swallowing. As observed in patients without cleft, impairment of dynamic function of the tube to relieve negative middle ear pressure may also be one of the causes for the development of OME in cleft palate.

The present study confirmed that middle ear disease is not affected by the type or laterality of clefts, nor by velopharyngeal insufficiency, presumably because a palatal cleft causes a similar degree of organic or functional impairment bilaterally in the eustachian tubes.

As OME in cleft palate patients shares many pathogenic factors with those observed in non-cleft patients, its treatment should consist primarily of ventilation of the middle ear as in ordinary OME.

References

Bluestone CD (1971) Eustachian tube obstruction in the infant with cleft palate. Ann Otol Rhinol Laryngol 80 (Supply 2): 1–30

Dickson DR (1976) Anatomy of the normal and cleft palate eustachian tube. Ann Otol Rhinol Laryngol 85 (Suppl 25): 25–29

Falk B, Magnuson B (1984) Eustachian tube closing failure. Occurrence in patients with cleft palate and middle ear disease. Arch Otolaryngol 110: 11–14

Fara M, Dvorak J (1970) Abnormal anatomy of the muscles of palatopharyngeal closure in cleft palates. Plast Reconstr Surg 46: 488–497

Kriens O (1975) Anatomy of the velopharyngeal area in cleft palate. Clin Plast Surg 2: 261–283

Latham RA, Long RE, Latham EA (1980) Cleft palate velopharyngeal musculature in a five-month-old infant: A three dimensional histological reconstruction. Cleft Palate J 17: 1–16

Mitoma T, Honjo I, Ushiro K, Tashima K (1985) Endoscopic findings of the pharyngeal orifices of the eustachian tube in cleft palates. Pract Otol (Kyoto) 78: 345–351 (in Japanese with English abstract)

Mitoma T (1986) Middle ear diseases in cleft palates. Pract Otol (Kyoto)79: 1413–1422 (in Japanese with English abstract)

Okazaki N, Honjo, I, Matsui H, Ushiro K, Nozoe T (1980) Middle ear disease in cleft palate children. Jibi Inkoka 52: 471–474 (in Japanese with English abstract)

Paulsen JW (1964) Studies on the hearing and the tubal function in a series of children with cleft palates (Preliminary report) Acta Otolaryngol Suppl 188: 36–44

Sataloff J, Fraser M (1952) Hearing loss in children with cleft palates. Arch Otolaryngol 55: 61–64

Spriestersbach DC, Lierle DM, Moll KL, Prather WF (1962) Hearing loss in children with cleft palates. Plast Reconstr Surg 30: 366–347

Surina I, Jagr J (1979) Action potentials of levator and tensor muscles in patients with cleft palates. Acta Chir Plast 11: 21–30

Chapter 9
Eustachian Tube in Chronic Otitis Media and Cholesteatoma

Disorders of the eustachian tube in chronic otitis media (COM) or cholesteatoma have long been regarded as an important problem. However, the question of how eustachian tube dysfunction affects the clinical course of middle ear disease and the prognosis of ear surgery have not been fully elucidated despite a large number of studies (Holmquist 1968; Andreasson and Harris 1979; Bluestone et al. 1979). Based on extensive experience in ear surgery, Sheehy (1981) contended that preoperative examination of the eustachian tube is unnecessary. At present, however, we lack sufficient information to evaluate the validity of this rather challenging opinion.

The vagueness of the relation between the eustachian tube and chronic ear disease is partly due to the method of examining tubal function. Simple tests such as tubal inflation by Politzer's or Valsalva's maneuver, which have been employed by clinicians, may obscure the exact connection between them. For the purpose of obtaining basic data on the relation between the eustachian tube and ear disease, several objective tests for tubal function were employed in the present study, and overall tubal functions were evaluated with regard to the prognosis of ear surgery. In addition, examination of the middle ear, especially around the tympanic orifice of the tube, were made during surgery to identify any disorder in the ear affecting eustachian tube function.

Attempts were made to answer the following questions: (a) How is the eustachian tube impaired in patients with COM? (b) what is the prognosis of tympanoplasty in patients with poor tubal function? (c) what are the essential tests for tubal function in predicting the result of tympanoplasty?

The formation of cholesteatoma has also been thought to be closely related to tubal dysfunction or to be a sequela of OME. Problems to be solved in this connection are: (a) How is the eustachian tube impaired in patients with cholesteatoma: and (b) how is the eustachian tube related to the pathogenesis of cholesteatoma?

9.1 Eustachian Tube Function in COM

There are already a number of studies concerning the eustachian tube in COM. Among them, Flisberg (1966), Holmquist (1969), and Sato et al. (1984) reported

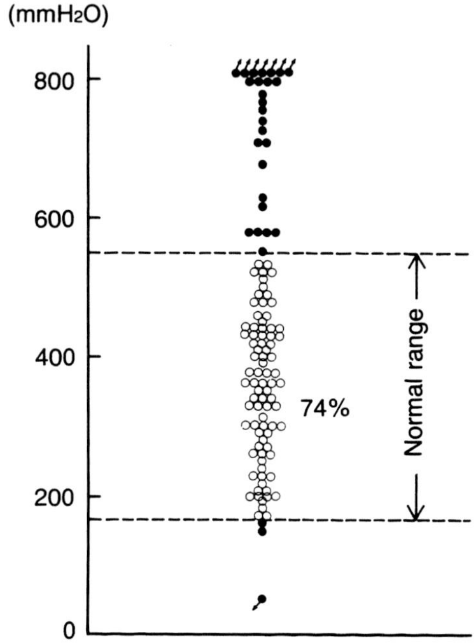

Fig. 9.1. Opening pressure of eustachian tube in chronic otitis media (111 ears)

that the results of the negative pressure test for tubal function were impaired in COM patients. In the present study, ventilatory and clearance functions of the eustachian tube were studied in a large number of COM ears, and overall evaluation of tubal function in COM was made to determine its correlation with surgical findings and prognosis of the ear.

9.1.1 Stenosis of Eustachian Tube and COM

The study included 111 unoperated ears with COM. The patients ranged in age from 5 to 75 years. The opening pressure of the eustachian tube in COM was normal (165–545 mmH_2O) in 74% of these patients (Fig. 9.1). Although the pressure was high in 23% of the patients, only 6% showed stenosis of the tube, whereby the tube did not open even when the middle ear pressure reached 800 mmH_2O. Thus, organic obstruction of the tube is fairly uncommon in COM.

Among the dynamic tests of the tube during swallowing, the results of the positive pressure test were good in 77% of 111 patients with COM (Fig. 9.2). This also indicated that no marked obstruction of the eustachian tube was present in COM. By contrast, the results of the negative pressure test were poor in almost half (47%) of the COM patients. Though impairment in relieving negative pressure was not as frequent as in OME, disturbance of the tube's ability to equalize negative middle ear pressure was regarded as a characteristic feature in COM patients.

Next, the clearance function of the eustachian tube was examined by means of the dye test. This function was normal in 66% of the ears examined (Fig. 9.3),

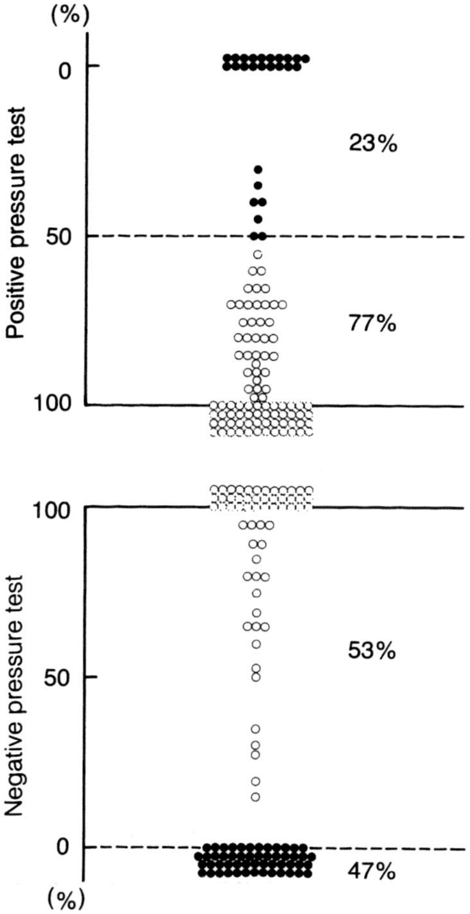

9.2

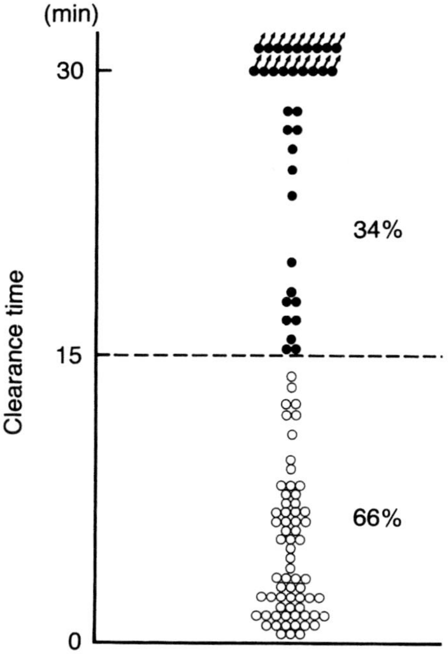

9.3

Fig. 9.2. Dynamic ventilatory function of eustachian tube in chronic otitis media (111 ears)

Fig. 9.3. Clearance function of eustachian tube in chronic otitis media (100 ears)

while it was severely impaired in 18 ears (18%). Among these 18 ears, however, obstruction of the tympanic orifice of the tube by granulation of marked edema was found in seven of the eight operated ears, suggesting that this impairment is not caused by the tube itself but is secondary to COM.

Thus, the patency of the eustachian tube in COM was unexpectedly good, and pathological conditions such as stenosis of the tube were uncommon. However, the ability to relieve negative middle ear pressure was impaired in about half of the patients.

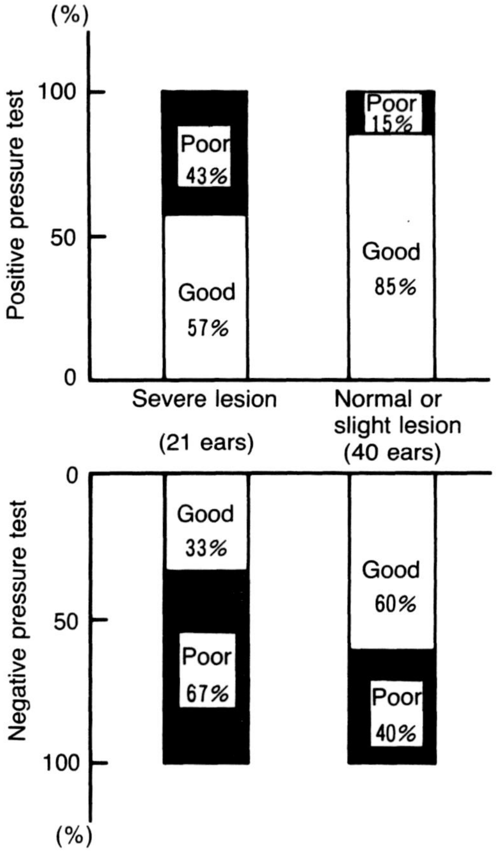

Fig. 9.4. Relation between lesions of tympanic orifice of eustachian tube and ventilatory function (61 ears)

9.1.2 Surgical Findings of Ear and Eustachian Tube Function

Next, the relation between inflammatory lesions around the tubal orifice and function of the tube was evaluated. These middle ear lesions were classified into two groups: severe lesion with polyp, granulation, or marked edema around the tympanic orifice of the tube, and minor lesion with only edema.

The results of the positive and negative pressure tests were poor in patients with severe lesions at the orifice, while in patients with slight or no lesions, ventilatory function of the tube was relatively good (Fig. 9.4). Impairment of the clearance function was also more frequent (48%) in patients with severe lesions at the orifice than in those with slight or no lesions (Fig. 9.5).

Next, the inflammatory lesions in the middle ear were examined with respect to the function of the eustachian tube. As shown in Fig. 9.6, overall function of the eustachian tube assessed by the three tests was graded from 1 to 4 according to the degree of impairment. It was found that the tubal impairment was proportional to the degree of lesions around the tympanic orifice in the ear. In the case of grade 1 impairment, a tympanic lesion was found in about two-thirds of the ears tested, while in grade 4 impairment it was noted in 90%. From these

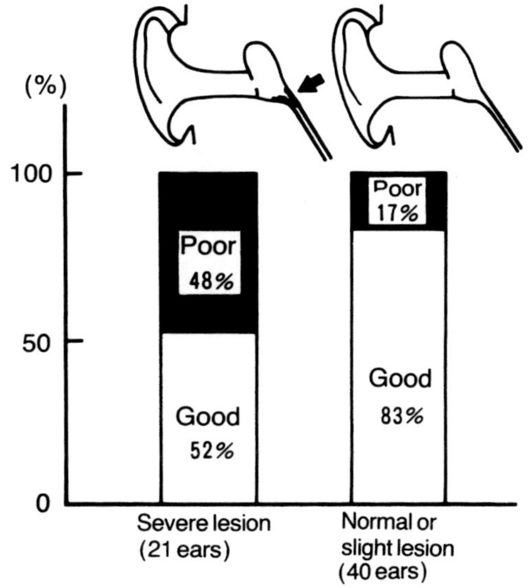

Fig. 9.5. Relation between lesions of tympanic orifice of eustachian tube and clearance function (61 ears)

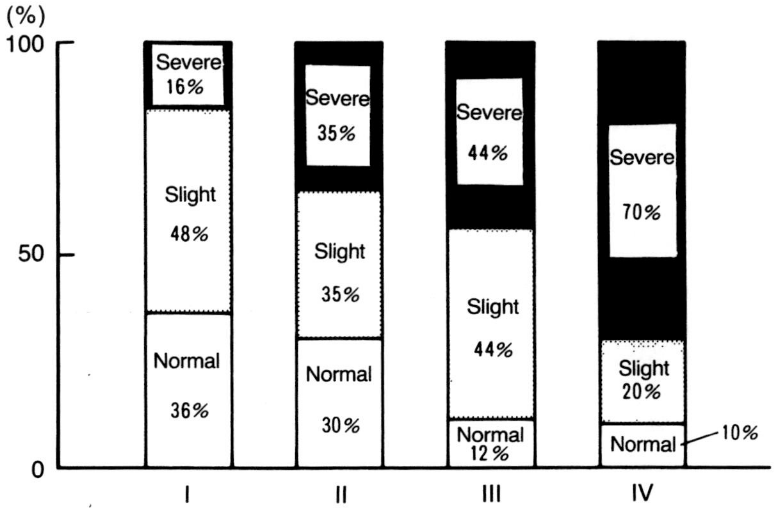

Fig. 9.6. Relation between eustachian tube function and lesions of tympanic orifice. *I* All tests (positive pressure, negative pressure, clearance tests) good, *II* only one test good, *III* two tests poor, *IV* all tests poor

results, an inflammatory or organic disorder around the tubal orifice of the ear should be taken into account when COM patients show significant impairment of eustachian tube function.

Impairment of ciliary clearance in COM was considered to be mainly caused by inflammation in the middle ear cavity. Since the inflammatory lesions in the ear can be controlled by ear surgery, improvement of both ventilatory and ciliary function of the tube after surgery can be expected.

Table 9.1. Eustachian tube function in chronic otitis media (100 ears)

Group	Positive pressure test	Negative pressure test	Clearance test	Ears	Comprehensive evaluation
I	Good	Good	Good	43	Good 66%
IIa	Good	Good	Poor	8	
IIb	Good	Poor	Good	15	
IIIa	Good	Poor	Poor	8	Poor 34%
IIIb	Poor	Poor	Good	8	
IV	Poor	Poor	Poor	18	

9.1.3 Integrated Evaluation of Eustachian Tube Function

The results of the three major tests for eustachian tube function are summarized in Table 9.1. As mentioned before, overall test results from 100 ears were divided into four groups according to the degree of impairment with two subclassifications in groups 2 and 3. Good results in all tests were obtained in 43% of the ears; however, if the tubal function is judged to be generally good even when the results of one test are unsatisfactory, then 66% of the ears fall into the category of "good." By contrast, 18% of the ears showed poor results in all tests, indicating that impairment of the eustachian tube in COM is relatively uncommon.

These results suggest that disturbance of the eustachian tube does not play a major role in COM, at least after establishment of the pathological condition of the ear disease. Since COM is always accompanied by perforation of the eardrum, the middle ear is always ventilated via the external ear canal. This ventilation may well result in normalization of the eustachian tube, except in cases with a marked inflammatory lesion at the tympanic orifice of the tube.

9.1.4. Summary

The results of ventilatory and clearance functions of the tube in 111 COM ears were as follows.

a) The opening pressure was normal in about 80% of the ears, and the dynamic function to relieve positive middle ear pressure was also satisfactory, suggesting that tubal obstruction in COM is rather rare. Results of the negative pressure test, however, were poor in nearly half of the ears. The clearance function of the tube was good in about 70%.
b) A close relation between middle ear lesion at the tympanic orifice of the tube and impairment of tubal function suggested tubal dysfunction caused by chronic inflammation in the ear.
c) If eustachian tube function was judged to be good when the results of all tests (positive and negative pressure tests and clearance test), or all except one test, were good, almost two-thirds of COM patients were judged to have good tubal function.

9.2 Effect of Eustachian Tube Function on Prognosis of Tympanoplasty

Tympanoplasty performed on COM patients is still unsuccessful in some cases, and this failure is often ascribed to dysfunction in the eustachian tube. Since the eardrum is closed after tympanoplasty, prognosis of ear surgery in patients with impaired ability of the tube to relieve negative pressure becomes problematic.

The relation between the results of tympanoplasty and the ventilatory function of the tube has been studied by many investigators. Among the dynamic function tests of the tube, the negative pressure test was often used as an index of the tubal function after tympanoplasty. Holmquist (1968), Siedentop et al. (1968), and Mackinnon (1970) found a positive correlation between the test results of negative pressure equalization and prognosis of ear surgery.

In the present study, the results of tympanoplasty were evaluated by both ventilatory and clearance functions of the tube, and overall test results of the tube were analyzed in relation to the clinical course after ear surgery.

9.2.1 Eustachian Tube Function and Results of Tympanoplasty

The results of ear surgery were judged to be satisfactory when disappearance of otorrhea, closure of the eardrum, and hearing improvement were obtained. In this study, hearing was judged to have improved when the average hearing level increased to more than 15 dB, the air-bone gap became less than 20 dB, or the hearing level became less than 40 dB. Forty ears with COM were evaluated 4–12 months after initial tympanoplasty (retroauricular approach, intact canal wall technique; 33 ears with type I and seven ears with modified type III with columella). Prognosis was judged to be bad, when more than one of the above three criteria was not satisfied.

Figure 9.7 shows the postoperative results in relation to the positive pressure test of the tube. Improvement in hearing after ear surgery was not satisfactory in patients showing poor results in the test. Other results such as aural discharge or

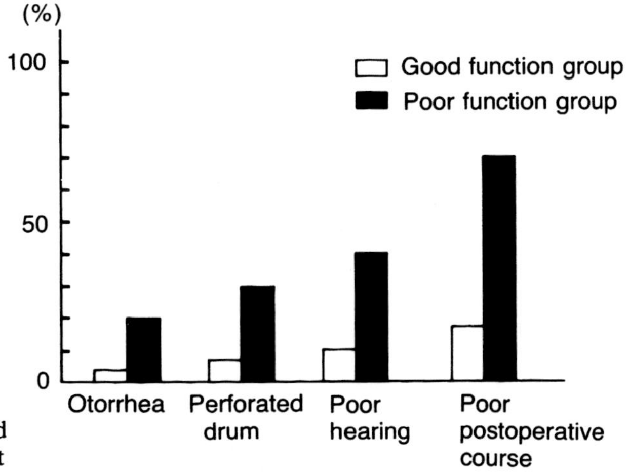

Fig. 9.7. Relation between outcome of tympanoplasty and results of positive pressure test

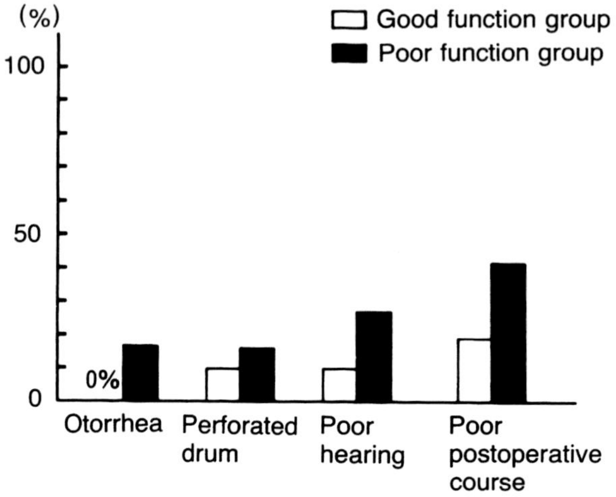

Fig. 9.8. Relation between outcome of tympanoplasty and results of negative pressure test

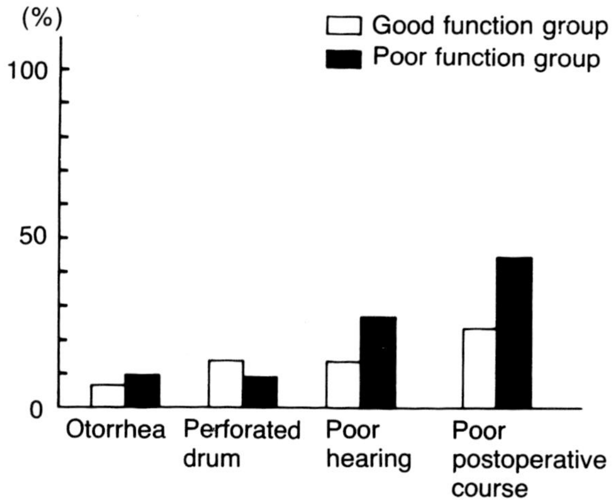

Fig. 9.9. Relation between outcome of tympanoplasty and clearance function

perforation of the eardrum were also correlated to the impaired function of the tube in the positive pressure test. The overall clinical course after tympanoplasty was also significantly worse when the results of this test were poor.

Figure 9.8 shows the relation between the results of the negative pressure test and postoperative findings of the ear. Contrary to expectation, there was no correlation between the results of this test and prognosis of ear surgery, except for the factor of hearing improvement. Thus, the negative pressure test appears to be of little value in determining the prognosis of tympanoplasty.

Figure 9.9 shows the relation between the clearance function of the tube and the postoperative course. The clearance function was related to neither the aural discharge nor perforation of the eardrum; it was associated with hearing improvement and the overall results after ear surgery.

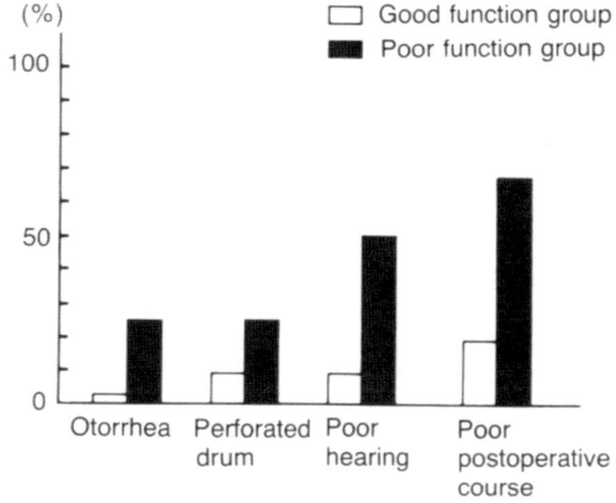

Fig. 9.10. Relation between outcome of tympanoplasty and overall eustachian tube function

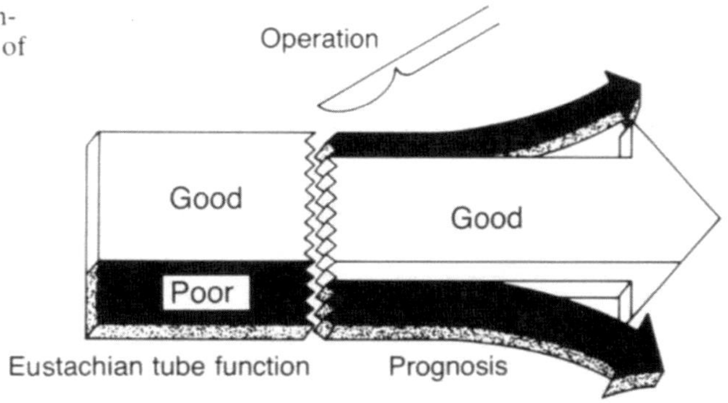

Fig. 9.11. Prognosis of tympanoplasty from standpoint of eustachian tube function

9.2.2 Tympanoplasty and Impaired Tubal Function

The overall function of the eustachian tube was regarded to be good when the results of more than two of three tests (positive and negative pressure tests and clearance test) were good. The postsurgical condition of the ear was compared between patients with good and poor tubal function. It was found that in the group with poor tubal function, disappearance of otorrhea, closure of the eardrum, and hearing gain were unsatisfactory. The overall results of ear surgery were also significantly poor in the group that had impaired function of the tube (Fig. 9.10).

Although a longer period of observation is necessary to reach a definitive conclusion, the present study indicated that the negative pressure test, which has been considered to be useful in estimating the prognosis of tympanoplasty, is of limited value; the positive pressure test or integrated evaluation of the tubal function is more useful for this purpose. As shown in Fig. 9.11, the prognosis of ear surgery largely depends on the preoperative function of the tube as examined by objective methods.

9.2.3 Summary

The influence of eustachian tube function on the results of ear surgery was studied. The results were as follows.

a) In general, eustachian tube function was closely correlated with the results of ear surgery, suggesting that tubal function plays an important role in the prognosis of tympanoplasty.
b) Among the tests for eustachian tube function, the negative pressure test, which had been regarded as being of prognostic value, was not correlated with the prognosis. The results of the positive pressure test could be correlated with the prognosis, and overall test results of tubal functions were also useful in determining the prognosis for tympanoplasty.

9.3 Eustachian Tube Function in Middle Ear Cholesteatoma

Reduction in the middle ear pressure due to obstruction or dysfunction of the eustachian tube may cause retraction of the pars flaccida of the eardrum, leading to the formation of cholesteatoma. Bluestone et al. (1978) considered that disorders of the eustachian tube were closely related to the pathogenesis of the cholesteatoma. Sano (1981) reported the formation of cholesteatoma in experimental animals by obstructing the eustachian tube.

In this study, the significance of the eustachian tube in the development of cholesteatoma, i.e., whether organic or functional obstruction of the tube is responsible for the development of cholesteatoma, was investigated. The function of the eustachian tube in cholesteatoma patients was examined before ear surgery with both conventional tests for tubal function and tests for closing failure of the tube. By comparing these test results with the surgical findings of the ear, the role of the eustachian tube in this disease was evaluated.

9.3.1 Eustachian Tube Impairment in Cholesteatoma

In 74 ears of 72 cholesteatoma patients, eustachian tube function was examined. According to the findings of the eardrum, cholesteatoma was divided into three groups as follows (Fig. 9.12): Retraction type (47 ears), a retraction or cholesteatoma mass in the pars flaccida or posterosuperior quadrant of the drum; perforation type (20 ears), a large defect or perforation mainly at the posteroinferior quadrant of the drum without abnormalities in the pars flaccida or posterosuperior quadrant; congenital type (7 ears), no abnormalities such as perforation or retraction in the eardrum but a mass in the middle ear seen through the drum.

The ventilatory function of the tube in retraction type cholesteatoma showed normal or reduced opening pressure in about 77% of the ears. Failure of tubal opening was observed in 11 ears (23%), while abnormally low pressure for tubal opening was noted in nine ears (19%; Fig. 9.13). Thus, mechanical obstruction of the eustachian tube is quite rare in retraction type cholesteatoma, which was the most common type of cholesteatoma in this study. The surgical findings indi-

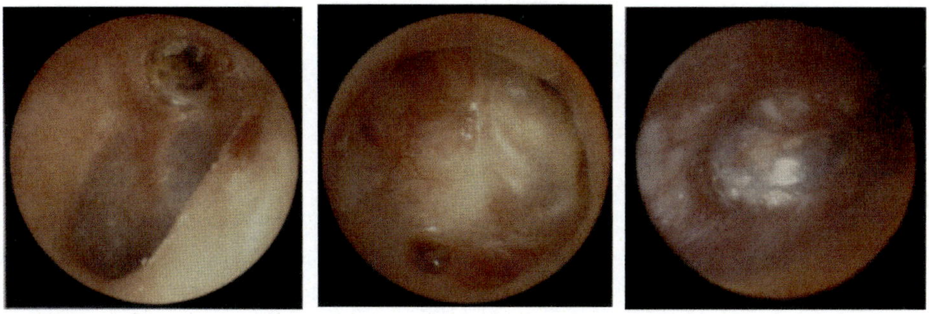

a, b c

Fig. 9.12a–c. Classification of middle ear cholesteatoma according to findings of tympanic membrane. **a** Retraction type; **b** Perforation type; **c** Congenital type

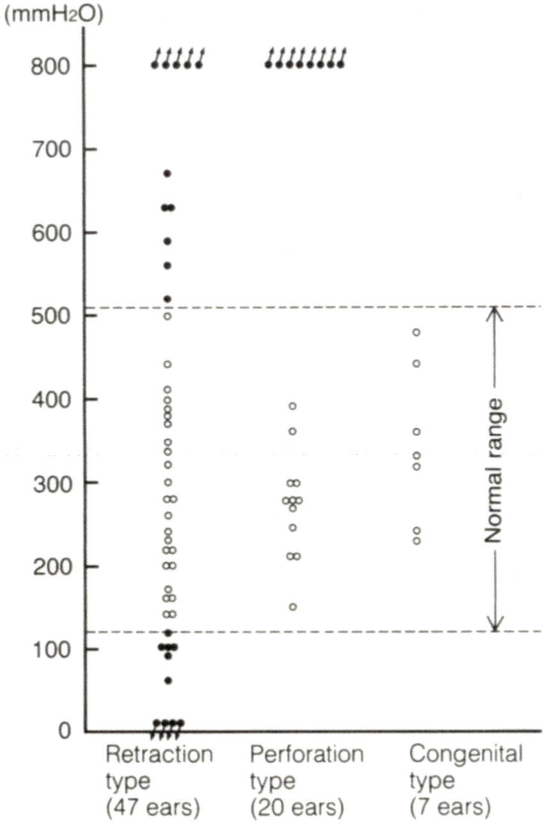

Fig. 9.13. Opening pressure of eustachian tube in middle ear cholesteatoma (74 ears)

cated that the tympanic orifice of the tube was normal in 70% (14 ears) of 20 patients with retraction type cholesteatoma. The percentage of normal findings of the orifice was significantly higher than in COM patients (Fig. 9.14).

In perforation type cholesteatoma, however, opening pressure of the tube was abnormally high in 40% (eight ears) of 20 cases. Relief of negative middle ear

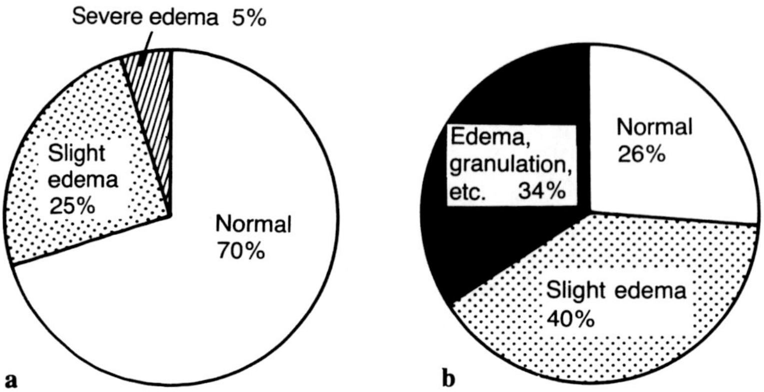

Fig. 9.14. **a** Lesions of tympanic orifice of eustachian tube in retraction type cholesteatoma (20 ears). **b** Lesions of tympanic orifice of eustachian tube in chronic otitis media (61 ears)

pressure was markedly impaired in about 80% of 20 ears with perforation type cholesteatoma, while positive pressure test results were poor in 45% (nine ears; Fig. 9.15). This type of cholesteatoma frequently showed an inflammatory lesion at the tympanic orifice of the tube, with about 60% of cases exhibiting granulation tissue around it.

The clearance function of the tube was good in patients with retraction type cholesteatoma (Fig. 9.16), while it was impaired in perforation type cholesteatoma, indicating that this tubal function is also closely correlated with the inflammatory lesions around the tympanic orifice.

These results suggest that mechanical obstruction of the eustachian tube is uncommon except for the tympanic lesion in perforation type cholesteatoma and that inflammation has little influence on the tubal function in retraction type cholesteatoma. The abnormally low opening pressure noted in retraction type cholesteatoma suggests closing failure of the tube in this type.

9.3.2 Pathogenesis of Cholesteatoma and Eustachian Tube

Functional obstruction of the eustachian tube has been considered to be a pathogenic factor in cholesteatoma. Based on the findings that the opening pressure of the tube in cholesteatoma children was either lower than or within the normal range and that the results of dynamic function of the tube was poor, Bluestone et al. (1978) proposed that functional obstruction of the tube causes high negative middle ear pressure, leading to the formation of cholesteatoma. In the present study, the opening pressure of the tube in retraction type cholesteatoma was normal or lower than normal, indicating increased patency of the tube in cholesteatoma patients. However, functional obstruction of the tube was relatively uncommon in this study because the results of the negative pressure test were good in about 60% of patients with retraction type cholesteatoma (Fig. 9.15), suggesting that this factor plays no significant role in the pathogenesis of cholesteatoma.

Fig. 9.15. Ventilatory function of eustachian tube in middle ear cholesteatoma (74 ears)

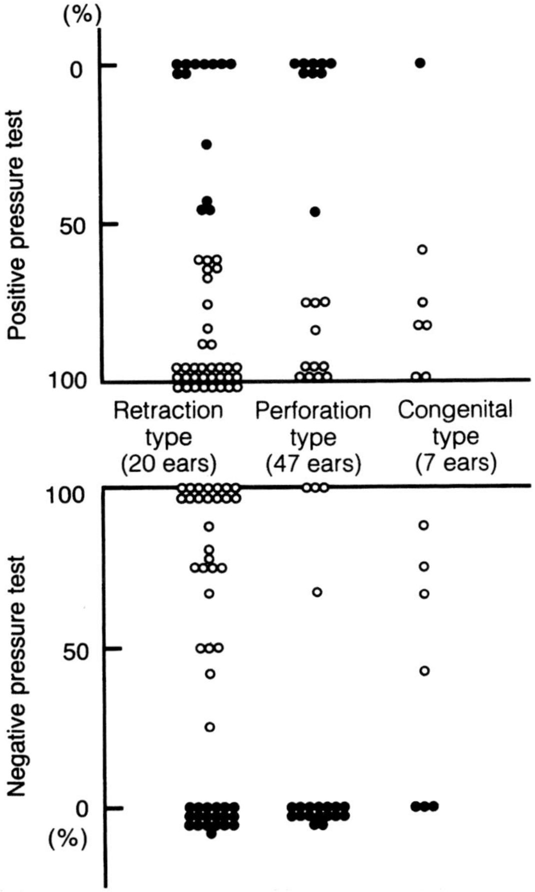

A marked lesion such as granulation or edema in the tympanic orifice of the tube, which might be related to the dysfunction of the tube, was observed both in perforated type cholesteatoma and in the retraction or congenital type cholesteatoma. Therefore, tubal dysfunction in cholesteatoma may be secondary to the inflammatory lesion around the tympanic orifice of the tube in the ear.

There is another opinion that cholesteatoma may develop in closing failure of the eustachian tube. Magnuson (1978) speculated that a negative middle ear pressure produced by sniffing causes retraction of the pars flaccida, leading to the formation of cholesteatoma. To evaluate this possibility, closing failure of the eustachian tube, permitting transmission of negative pressure to the middle ear by sniffing, was examined using manosonotubometry in 47 ears of retraction type cholesteatoma. Closing failure of the tube, as shown in Fig. 9.17, was noted only in about 26% of cases, indicating that the formation of negative middle ear pressure by sniffing may not be frequent (Fig. 9.18). This theory is based on the assumption that negative middle ear pressure caused by sniffing cannot be re-

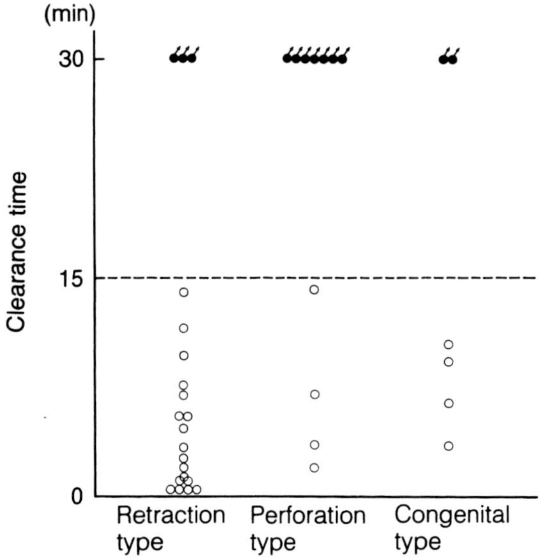

Fig. 9.16. Clearance function of eustachian tube in middle ear cholesteatoma (39 ears)

lieved once it has formed. However, the majority of patients were able to relieve negative middle ear pressure during swallowing. Therefore, sniffing cannot be regarded as a major pathogenetic factor in cholesteatoma.

In any event, the present study demonstrated that the pathogenesis of cholesteatoma cannot be ascribed simply to impaired patency of the eustachian tube; however, it is also difficult to explain on the basis of closing failure of the tube. A longitudinal study involving functional and morphological examinations is essential for further elucidation of the pathogenesis of cholesteatoma.

9.3.3 Summary

Eustachian tube function was examined in 78 ears with cholesteatoma. The results were as follows.

a) The opening pressure of the eustachian tube was normal or reduced in retraction type cholesteatoma, indicating the absence of organic obstruction of the tube.
b) The ventilatory function of the tube could be correlated to the surgical findings around the tubal orifice in the middle ear, suggesting that the tubal dysfunction in cholesteatoma may be secondary to chronic inflammation in the ear.
c) Closing failure of the tube was noted in about 26% of cases in retraction type cholesteatoma, suggesting that it plays no major role in the development of this disease.

9.4 Summary of Chapter

Eustachian tube function in COM as evaluated by ventilatory and clearance function tests revealed that obstruction of the tube is rather uncommon. Despite

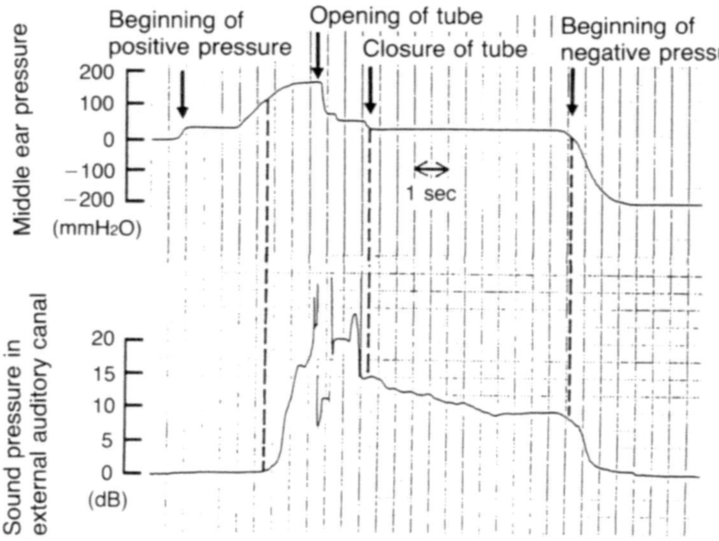

Fig. 9.17. Closing failure of eustachian tube by manosonotubometry

Fig. 9.18. Closing failure of eustachian tube in retraction type cholesteatoma (47 ears)

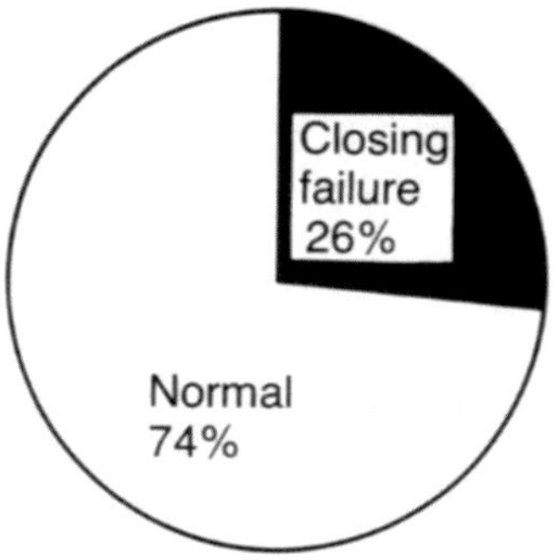

the long-standing concept that the tubal function in COM is impaired, it was found that middle ear ventilation through the eustachian tube is generally satisfactory.

When the prognosis of ear surgery was evaluated by closure of the eardrum, drying of the ear, and hearing improvement, it was found that the prognosis was not satisfactory in COM patients with poor function of the tube. Therefore, care should be taken with COM patients, one-third of whom have poor tubal function before surgery. However, impairment of tubal function was partly caused by chronic inflammation in the ear or obstruction of the tympanic orifice of the tube by granulation, which can be controlled by surgery. Although overall evaluation of tubal functions is desirable before ear surgery, examination of the ability to relieve positive middle ear pressure during swallowing was useful for estimating the prognosis of tympanoplasty. When relief of positive pressure was impaired, the operation was often unsuccessful.

Middle ear cholesteatoma appears to be closely related to the retraction pocket of the eardrum or a sequela of OME. Obstruction of the eustachian tube was rather uncommon in cholesteatoma, especially in the retraction type of cholesteatoma. On the other hand, perforation type cholesteatoma showed marked impairment of the ventilatory function of the tube and was closely correlated to the inflammatory lesion around the tympanic orifice of the tube. Thus, tubal dysfunction in this type was considered to be the result of inflammation due to the cholesteatoma. Although the eustachian tube tended to be patent in retraction type cholesteatoma, closing failure of the tube was not frequent in these patients. More detailed clinical and experimental investigations with respect to the eustachian tube are required for the study of pathogenesis of cholesteatoma.

References

Andreasson L, Harris S (1979) Middle ear mechanics and eustachian tube function in tympanoplasty. Acta Otolaryngol Suppl 360: 141–147

Bluestone CD, Cantekin EI, Beery QC, Stool SE (1978) Function of the eustachian tube related to surgical management of aquired aural cholesteatoma in children. Laryngoscope 88: 1155–1164

Bluestone CD, Cantekin EI, Douglas GS (1979) Eustachian tube function related to the results of tympanoplasty in children. Laryngoscope 89: 450–458

Flisberg K (1966) Ventilatory studies on the eustachian tube. A clinical investigation of cases with perforated ear drums. Acta Otolaryngol Suppl 219: 1–82

Holmquist J (1968) The role of the eustachian tube in myringoplasty. Acta Otolaryngol 66: 289–295

Holmquist J (1969) Eustachian tube function in patients with ear drum perforations following chronic otitis media. Acta Otolaryngol 68: 391–401

Mackinnon DM (1970) Relationship of pre-operative eustachian tube function to myringoplasty. Acta Otolaryngol 69: 100–106

Magnuson B (1978) Tubal closing failure in retraction type cholesteatoma and adhesive middle ear lesions. Acta Otolaryngol 86: 408–417

Sano S (1981) Experimental middle ear cholesteatoma. ORL Tokyo 24: 129–171 (in Japanese with English abstract)

Sato Y, Takahashi S, Imai A, Nakano Y (1984) Inflation-deflation tests in ears with tympanic membrane perforation. Jibi Inkoka 56: 411–416 (Japanese with English abstract)

Sheehy JL (1981) Testing eustachian tube function. Ann Otol Rhinol Laryngol 90: 562–564

Siedentop KH, Tardy ME, Hamilton LR (1968) Eustachian tube function. Arch Otolaryngol 88: 386–395. 1968

Chapter 10
Effects of Middle Ear Pressure on Hearing and Equilibrium

Hearing impairment due to abnormal middle ear pressure is often experienced in the case of eustachian tube obstruction or rapid changes in the environmental pressure as in diving or flying. On the other hand, hearing impairment in OME patients is known to be associated not only with a reduction in air conduction but also with a reduction in bone conduction, which can be relieved by treatment of OME. Thus, abnormal middle ear pressure appears to cause reversible bone conduction hearing loss. Fowler (1920) reported hearing impairment due to a reduction in the bone conduction of the low-tone range by application of pressure through the eustachian tube into the middle ear.

Changes in middle ear pressure are also known to affect equilibrium. Fukuda (1984; Japanese original published in 1957) reported that stepping deviation observed in OME patients disappeared after inflating the ear with air and thought this to be caused by the inner ear pressure change due to displacement of the eardrum and the stapes. Ingelstedt et al. (1974) also reported cases of nystagmus induced by pressure to the middle ear of normal subjects.

These clinical findings suggest that abnormalities in the middle ear pressure affect the functions of the cochlea and vestibule. The detailed mechanism of these effects, however, remains to be clarified. Questions to be elucidated in this study are: (a) Does negative middle ear pressure in OME impair bone-conduction hearing? (b) does bone-conduction hearing loss result from cochlear dysfunction? (c) does middle ear pressure affect equilibrium? and (d) does middle ear pressure also affect vestibular function?

10.1 Effect of Middle Ear Pressure on Hearing

In patients with OME, hearing can be affected not only by the negative middle ear pressure but also by fluid retained in the middle ear. The eardrum and middle ear ossicles may also influence hearing under negative middle ear pressure. These factors were eliminated as far as possible in the present study and the effects of middle ear pressure on bone-conduction hearing were evaluated clinically and experimentally.

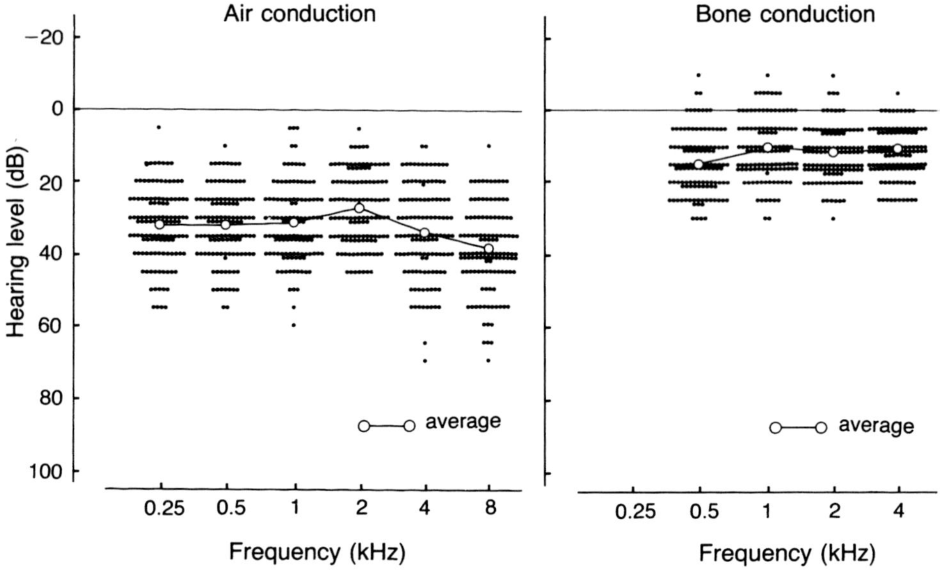

Fig. 10.1. Audiograms of OME patients (120 ears with OME children)

10.1.1 Hearing in Patients with OME

The general features of air- and bone-conduction hearing were studied in 120 ears of 97 children with OME (aged 5–15 years, mean 7.7 years). A Rion AA-63BN audiometer (bone-conduction receiver BR-41) was used. Air conduction was examined at six frequencies (250, 500, 1000, 2000, 4000 and 8000 Hz), and bone conduction at four frequencies (500, 1000, 2000, and 4000 Hz).

As shown in Fig. 10.1, average air-conduction hearing loss was about 30 dB in OME patients, while bone-conduction hearing loss was about 10 dB, with a notable reduction in the low-tone range of 500 Hz. Figure 10.2 shows hearing improvement after the treatment for OME. Air-conduction hearing improved markedly after tympanostomy tube insertion, and bone-conduction hearing also improved, mainly at 500 and 1000 Hz. This improvement in bone-conduction hearing, however, may be due to removal of the effusion after myringotomy as well as normalization of the middle ear pressure.

The incidence of bone-conduction hearing loss in OME patients and hearing improvement following myringotomy was examined in 83 ears of 72 OME patients (aged 6–49 years, mean 18.0 years). The normal range of bone-conduction hearing was determined in 42 ears of 21 normal controls (aged 14–36 years, mean 22.8 years). It was revealed that 34.9% (29 ears) of the ears with OME were below the normal range of bone-conduction hearing. After the treatment for OME, the percentage of ears with reduced bone conduction decreased to 21.7% (18 ears; Fig. 10.3).

The effect of myringotomy only on bone conduction was then evaluated without the removal of effusion. Fifty ears of 40 patients with OME were studied (aged 6–75 years, mean 26.4 years). To eliminate the errors of two measure-

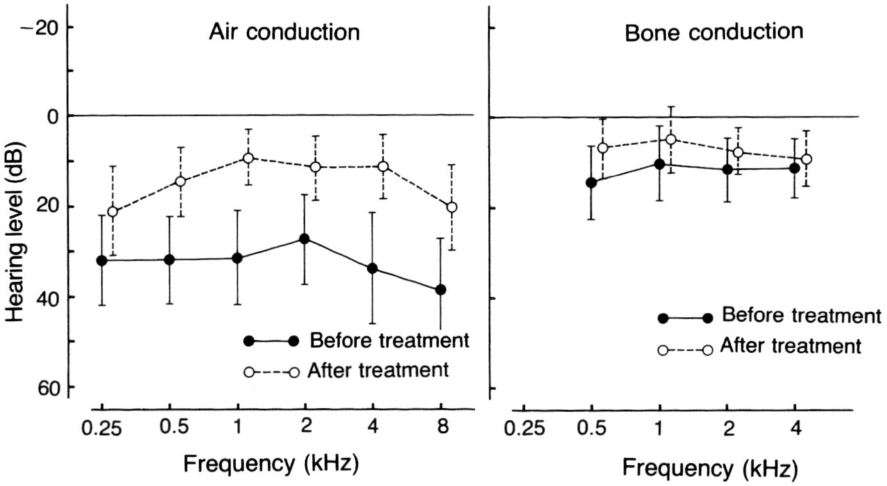

Fig. 10.2. Audiograms before and after tympanostomy tube insertion (120 ears with OME children). Means and 1 SD are plotted

ments before and after myringotomy, changes in bone-conduction hearing in OME were compared with those of 20 normal control ears measured twice. As shown in Fig. 10.4, changes in bone conduction after myringotomy were most notable at 500 Hz. Improvement in hearing at this frequency was observed in 22% (11 ears) of the subjects, which was significantly better than at other frequencies. Deterioration of bone-conduction hearing at 500 Hz was also noted in 10% of 50 subjects, but this was not significant compared with that at other frequencies. At 1000, 2000, and 4000 Hz, improvement and deterioration occurred almost equally, indicating no significant improvement after myringotomy.

Figure 10.5 shows the mean bone-conduction hearing of 11 ears (five ears with serous effusion and six with mucous effusion) which showed significant improvement after myringotomy. Improvement was most notable at 500 Hz, followed by 1000 Hz, while no improvement was observed at high frequencies of 2000 and 4000 Hz. This immediate improvement in bone conduction is considered to be due to relief from negative middle ear pressure by myringotomy. These findings were consistent with the previous finding that the improvement in bone conduction by treatment of OME was in the low-tone range.

10.1.2 Effect of Negative Middle Ear Pressure on Bone-Conduction Hearing

Apart from OME, changes in bone-conduction hearing by relief of negative middle ear pressure alone were studied in patients who showed type-C tympanograms. Bone conduction hearing was compared between ten ears in ten children (aged 6–14 years, mean 9.0 years) showing a type-C tympanogram (peak values −100 to −400 mmH_2O) and 20 normal ears in 13 children of the same age (6–12 years, mean 7.5 years) who showed a type-A tympanogram.

As presented in Fig. 10.6, the first group of children who had negative middle ear pressure showed reduced bone conduction only at 500 Hz compared with the

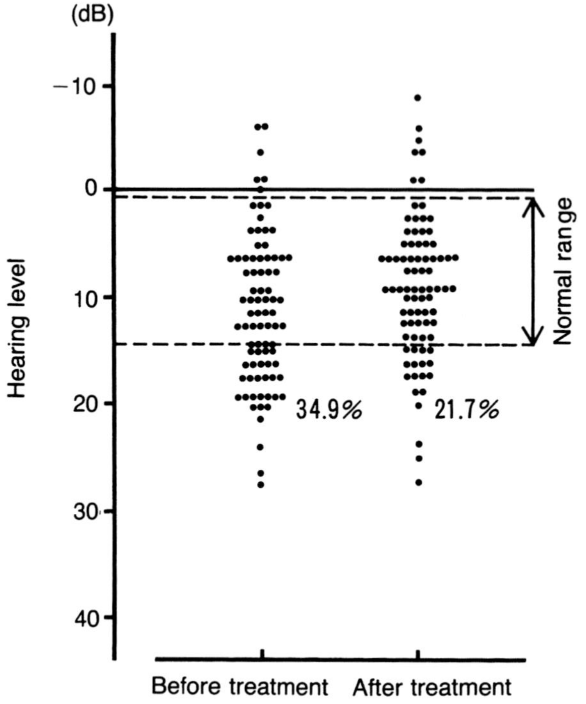

Fig. 10.3. Mean bone-conduction hearing levels before and after removal of middle ear effusion (50 ears with OME)

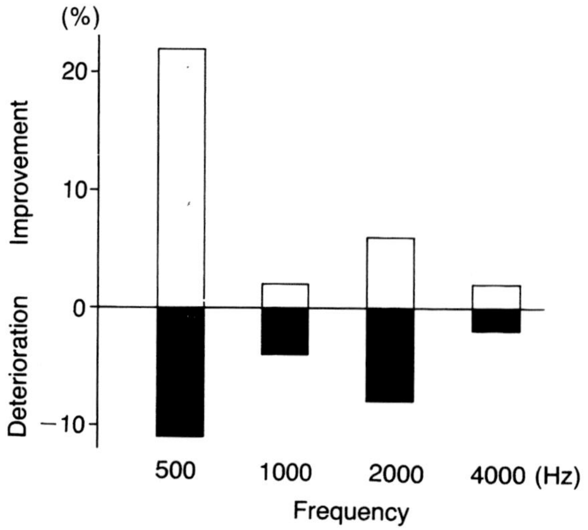

Fig. 10.4. Changes in bone conduction after myringotomy without removal of middle ear effusion (50 ears with OME)

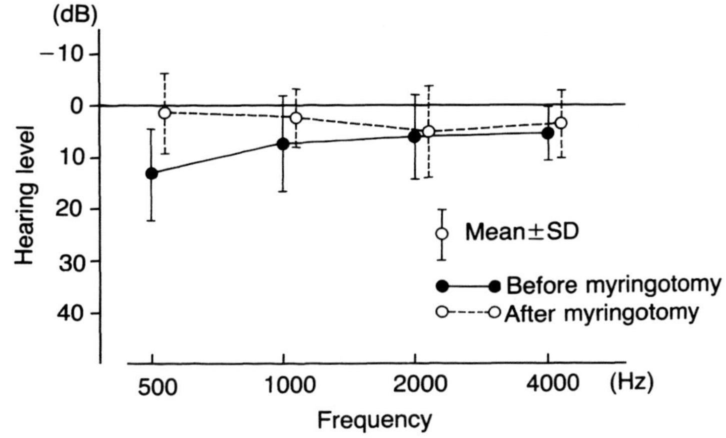

Fig. 10.5. Changes in bone conduction in 11 ears in which significant improvements were observed after myringotomy without removal of middle ear effusion

normal pressure group, similar to the findings in OME ears.

For the same purpose, bone-conduction hearing of 15 ears of 15 patients who had a perforated eardrum (aged 6–57 years, mean 27.8 years) was examined when a negative middle ear pressure of −300 or −500 mmH_2O was applied through the perforation. As shown in Fig. 10.7, the effect of negative middle ear pressure on bone-conduction hearing was greatest at 500 Hz, with an 8.5 dB reduction under −500 mmH_2O; at 1000 Hz, however, the reduction was only 3.5 dB.

10.2 Experimental Study on Effect of Middle Ear Pressure on Inner Ear Function

There have been several experimental studies on the effects of negative middle ear pressure on bone-conduction hearing. Using cats, Wever et al. (1942) concluded that the reduction in bone conduction measured by cochlear microphonics (CM) under negative middle ear pressure was caused by increased stiffness of the eardrum, since no reduction of CM was observed when the middle ear ossicles were interrupted. On the other hand, Sawashima (1957) and Tonndorf and Tabor (1960) observed a reduction in bone-conduction hearing after experimental closure of the round window and ascribed this reduction to impaired mobility of the round window.

In the present study, CM were measured in each cochlear turn of guinea pigs. Although sound stimulation was applied by air conduction, displacement of the eardrum and the ossicles was minimized by applying equal pressure to both the middle and external ear canal according to the method by Rahm et al. (1958). Therefore, the results are thought to reflect cochlear function, including that of the inner ear windows, and indicate the effects of negative middle ear pressure on bone-conduction hearing.

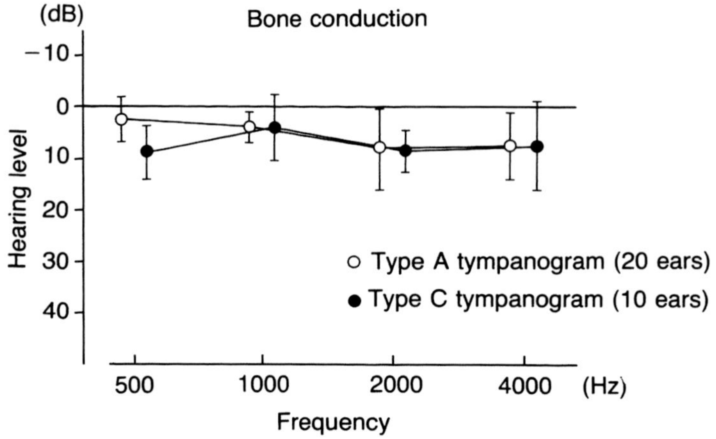

Fig. 10.6. Comparison of bone conduction between ten ears with type-A tympanograms and 20 ears with type C tympanograms

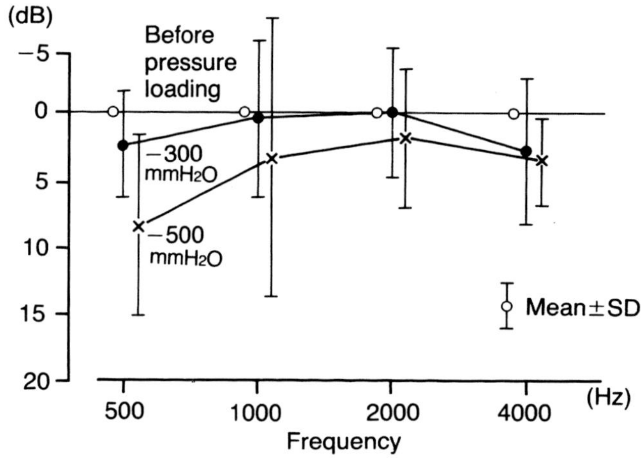

Fig. 10.7. Effect of middle ear negative pressure on bone conduction (15 ears with perforation of the eardrum)

Twenty-three guinea pigs were anesthetized with pentobarbital, and muscle relaxant (pancuronium bromide) was administered. CM were recorded from each cochlear turn during stimulation with air-conducted pure tones of 500, 1000, 2000, and 40000 Hz (50–90 dB soundpressure level; Fig. 10.8).

As shown in Fig. 10.9, CM decreased rapidly following the application of negative pressure to the middle ear. This reduction continued while the negative middle ear pressure was sustained but promptly recovered after the pressure was relieved. Negative middle ear pressure, therefore, was considered to have a reversible effect on the cochlear function. The reduction in CM was also found to be proportional to the negative pressure applied to the middle ear (Fig. 10.10).

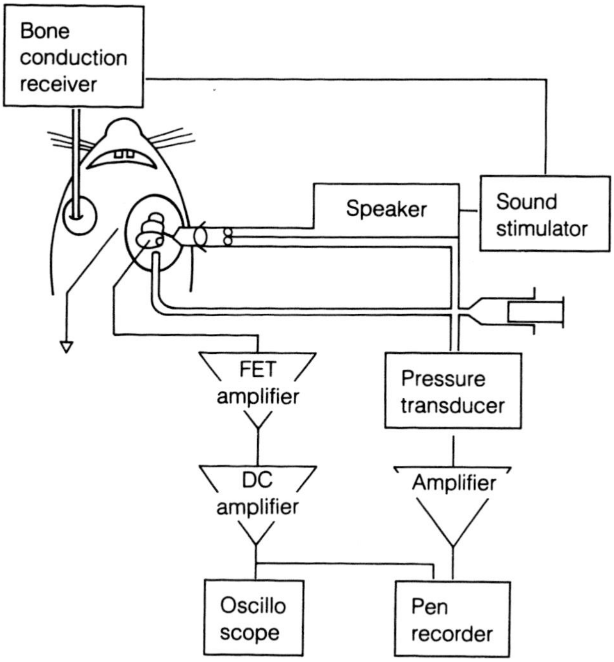

Fig. 10.8. Scheme of CM measurement

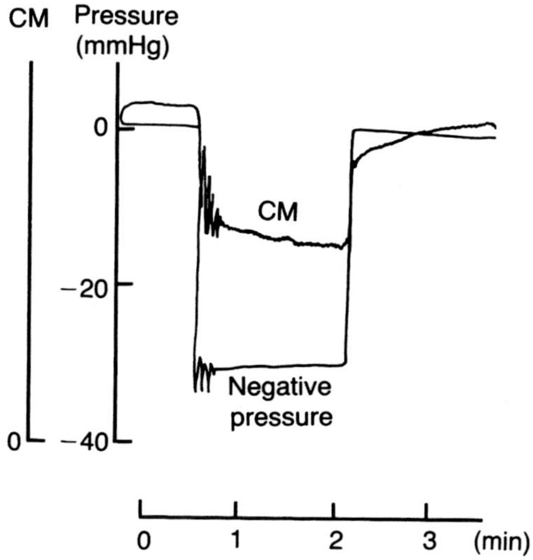

Fig. 10.9. Reduction of CM amplitude by application of negative pressure in middle ear and external auditory canal

Of the CM of each cochlear turn, the CM from the basal and apical turns are shown in Fig. 10.11. CM was reduced at all frequencies under negative middle ear pressure. In the basal turn, the reduction in the low-tone range was notable but that in the high-tone range was slight. On the other hand, at the apical turn, reduction in the middle- and high-tone ranges was noted as well as in the low-tone range. The reduction in CM was 2–9 dB, which was comparable with that in bone-conduction hearing in humans (5–10 dB).

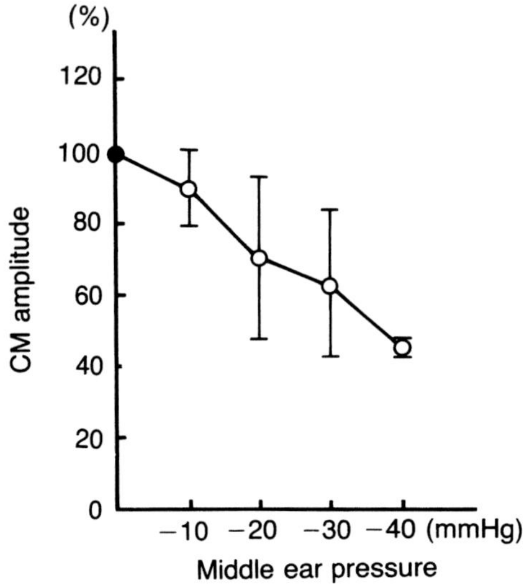

Fig. 10.10. Relation between CM amplitude and pressure in middle ear and external auditory canal

Since no displacement of the eardrum was noted in any of the experimental animals, the effects of pressure on the eardrum and the middle ear ossicles were negligible. Reduction in bone-conduction hearing, therefore, appears to be due to impairment of cochlear function, resulting from changes in the stiffness of the inner ear windows or in the inner ear pressure.

10.2.1 Summary

The effect of negative middle ear pressure on bone-conduction hearing was studied in 65 humans (75 ears) and 23 guinea pigs. The results were as follows.
a) In humans, negative middle ear pressure observed in OME patients caused a reduction in bone conduction at the low frequency of 500 Hz.
b) In guinea pigs, CM under negative middle ear pressure showed a temporary reduction at 500 and 1000 Hz, suggesting that bone-conduction hearing loss in OME patients is due to cochlear dysfunction.

10.3 Effects of Middle Ear Pressure on Equilibrium

Abnormal middle ear pressure may affect the inner ear via a labyrinthine fistula, but even in patients without a fistula the middle ear pressure is known to cause vestibular dysfunction. However, the mechanism of how it affects the vestibular function has not been clarified. Therefore, vestibular function was evaluated with respect to the sway of the head and the center of gravity in humans.

A position sensor (C1373, Hamamatsu Photonics, Hamamatsu, Japan) was used to examine the head sway, and a stabilometer (G1800, Anima, Tokyo, Japan) was used for evaluation of swaying of the center of gravity. Swaying was recorded in the standing position with the eyes open and closed for 60 s each, and the data were analyzed with a personal computer (PC9801, NEC, Tokyo, Japan) after A-D conversion.

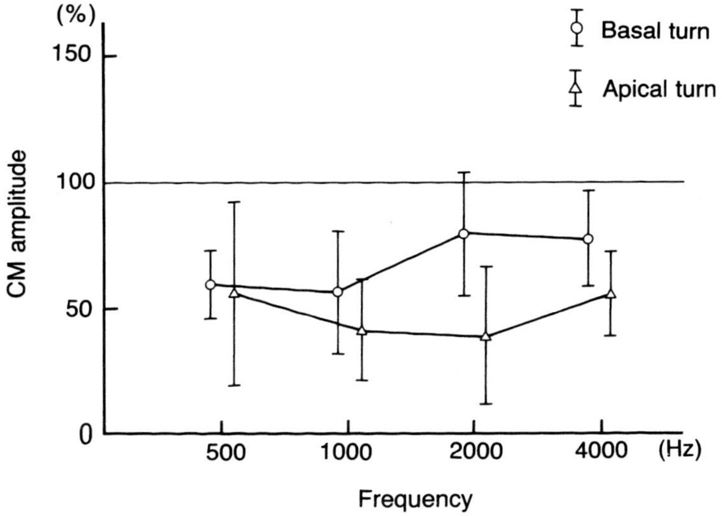

Fig. 10.11. Change in CM amplitude under negative pressure in middle ear and external auditory canal

The mean of 1200 position coordinates of the head and the center of gravity obtained during 60 s was regarded as the center of sway of the head and body. The extent of the shift of this center to the affected or normal side with the eyes closed as compared with the eyes open (deviation, D) was measured. Sways of the head and the center of gravity were evaluated according to the deviation ratio (D/R %), or the percentage of the deviation (D) to the amplitude of sways measured with the eyes closed (R; Fig. 10.12).

10.3.1 Equilibrium in Patients with OME

In 25 patients with unilateral OME, the sways of the head and the center of gravity were evaluated by the method described above before and after myringotomy. The shift of the center of sway with the eyes closed to the affected side was regarded as positive and that to the normal side as negative. With the eyes closed, both the head and the center of the gravity shifted slightly to the affected side (D/R +4.29% ± 22.27% for the head and +1.52% ± 14.00% for the center of gravity) before the treatment, but slightly to the normal side (D/R −7.00% ± 19.73% for the head and −3.90% ± 14.31% for the center of gravity) after treatment for OME (Fig. 10.13).

These shifts of the center were more notable in the head, and the shift of the head deviation from the affected side before the treatment to the normal side after the treatment was significant (paired sample Student's *t*-test $P < 0.01$).

10.3.2 Pressure Change in Middle Ear or External Ear Canal on Equilibrium

To analyze the factors responsible for the shift of the head and the center of gravity, the effects of positive and negative middle ear pressure on equilibrium

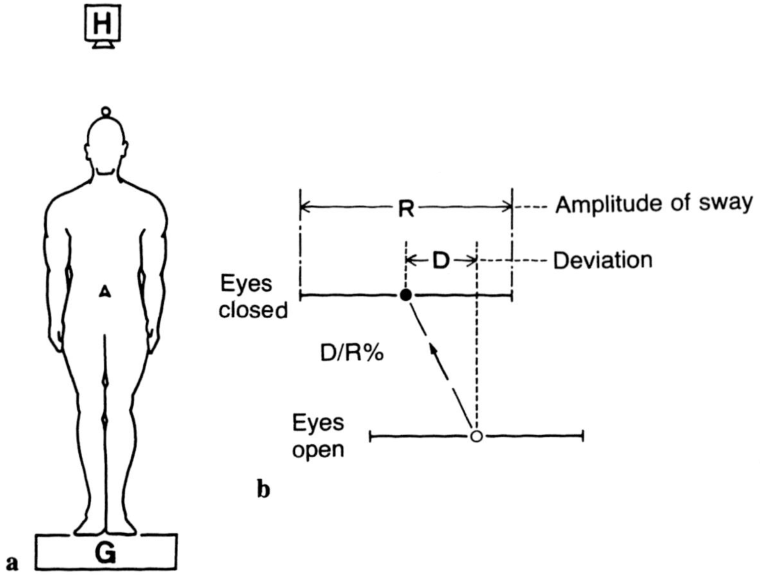

Fig. 10.12. **a** Measurement of head and body sway. **b** Calculation of deviation ratio. *G* Platform for measurement of sway of body's center of gravity, *H* infrared camera for measuring head movement

were studied in ten adults in the convalescent stage of OME. Through a tympanostomy tube, pressure of ±150 mmH_2O was applied to the middle ear. As shown in Fig. 10.14, the head deviation shifted to the opposite side (D/R −11.91% ±25.11%) when a positive pressure was applied, but to the side of pressure (+12.32% ± 22.34%) when the pressure was negative.

Next, the effect of external auditory canal pressure on equilibrium was examined in normal ears with an intact eardrum (15 individuals). A positive or negative pressure of ±300 mmH_2O was applied to the external auditory canal (Fig. 10.15). The head deviation shifted to the side of the pressure (D/R +10.76% ± 17.96%) when the pressure was positive but to the opposite side (D/R −11.65% ± 15.80%) when it was negative. The direction of the head deviation by application of pressure to the external ear canal was the opposite of that when the pressure was applied to the middle ear.

Figure 10.16 shows changes in the sway of the head expressed as the arithmetic mean while positive and negative pressures were applied alternately for 20 s each to the ear canal. The head shifted to the side of the pressure when the pressure was positive, and to the opposite side when it was negative. This shift occurred not only when the pressure changed, but continued while the pressure was sustained. The same test was performed in a patient in whom inner ear function was completely destroyed by a temporal bone fracture. As shown in Fig. 10.17, no significant shift of the head was observed despite positive or negative pressure in the external auditory canal.

The present study in OME patients revealed that the direction of the deviation of the head changes significantly from the affected side to the normal

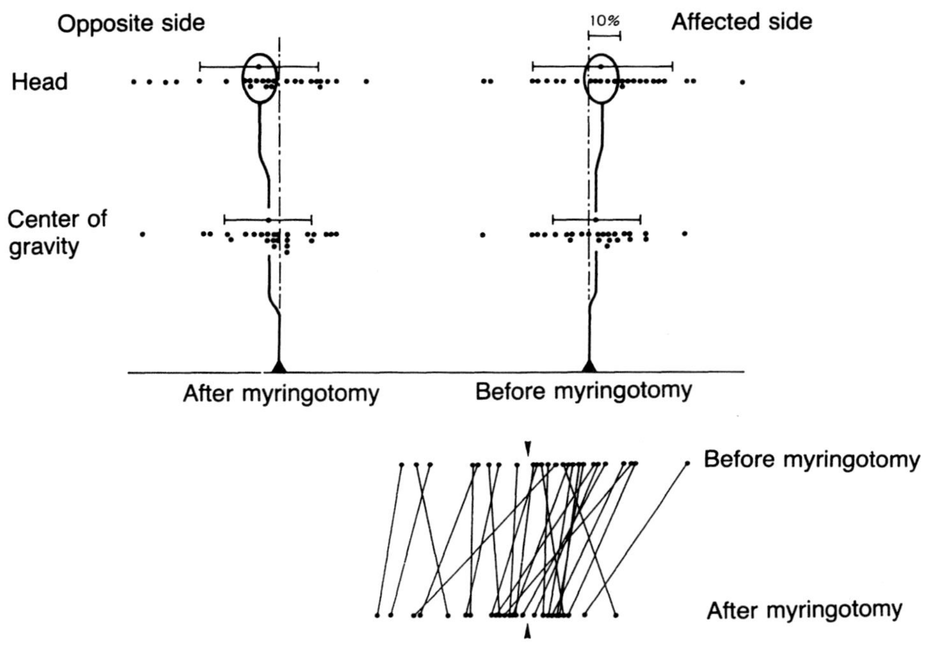

Fig. 10.13. Deviation ratio before and after myringotomy ($n = 25$, $t = 3.65$, $P < 0.01$)

side with resolution of OME. In addition, the direction of the head deviation was reversed under conditions of pressure of the middle ear and of the external ear canal. These findings suggest that such deviation is mediated by the middle or inner ear system.

10.4 Experimental Study on Effects of Middle Ear Pressure on Vestibular System

To examine whether changes in the middle ear pressure affect vestibular function, the activities of the vestibular nerve were examined in cats.

10.4.1 Effect of Middle Ear Pressure on Vestibular Nerve

Thirteen cats anesthetized with α-chloralose were examined. Figure 10.18 is a schematic diagram of the experiment. The pharyngeal orifice of the eustachian tube was blocked and pressure was applied to the middle ear through a perforation in the eardrum. The middle ear pressure was monitored with a pressure transducer (P23ID, Gould H.B., CA, USA) and was increased or reduced by a maximum of about 800 mmH_2O.

The cats were fixed in a stereotaxic apparatus, which was mounted on a turntable that allowed three-dimensional rotation. The head was tilted 21° from the horizontal plane to achieve maximum effective stimulation of the semicircular

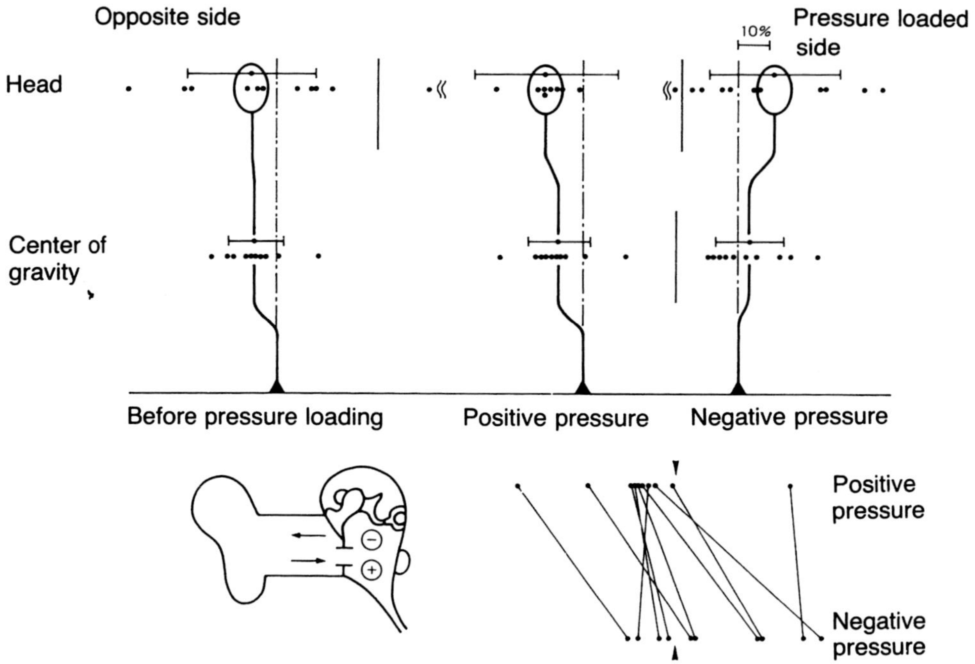

Fig. 10.14. Changes in deviation ratio according to middle ear pressure ($n = 10$, $t = 3.90$, $P < 0.01$)

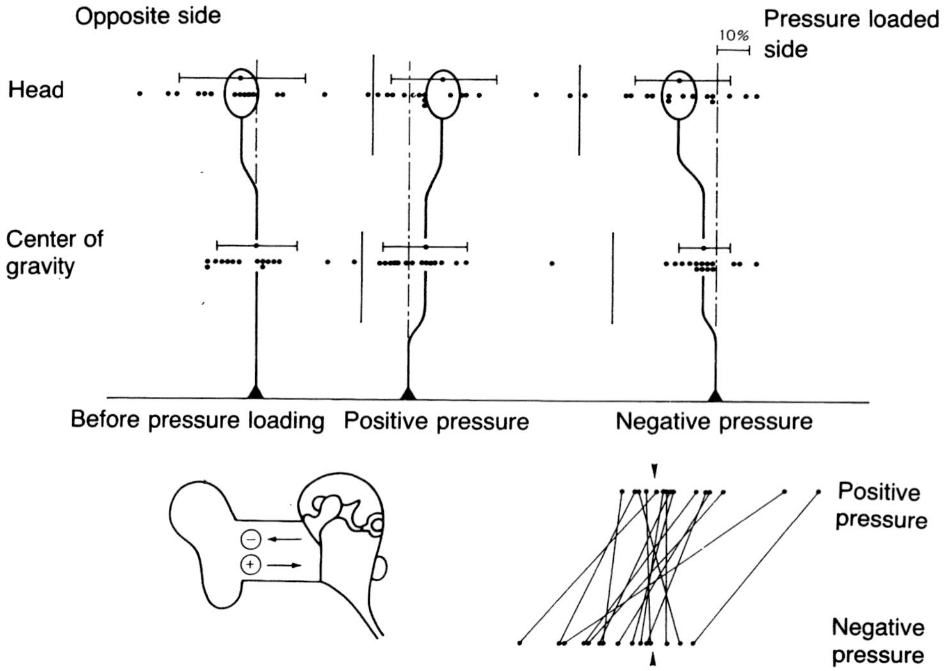

Fig. 10.15. Changes in deviation ratio according to the external auditory canal pressure ($n = 15$, $t = 3.84$, $P < 0.01$)

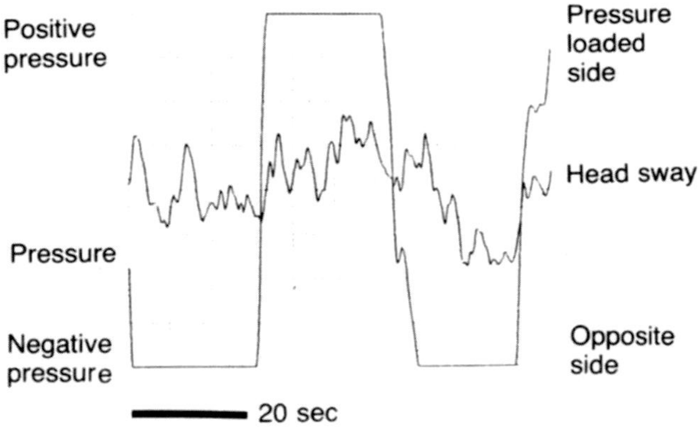

Fig. 10.16. Head sway while positive or negative pressure was applied to the external auditory canal

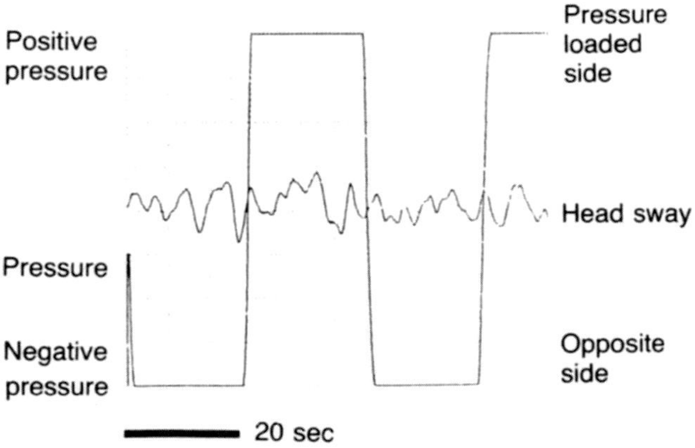

Fig. 10.17. Head sway of a patient whose inner ear function was suppressed by a temporal bone fracture. No significant shift was observed despite positive or negative pressure in external auditory canal

canals. Intra-axonal recording of vestibular nerve activity was made with a glass microelectrode filled with 3 *M* KCl.

The position of the vestibular nerve (0.5 mm caudal to the center of the genu of the facial nerve, 5–6 mm lateral to the median line, and 0.5–1.5 mm below the floor of the fourth ventricle) was confirmed under a microscope following the brain atlas of Snider and Niemer.

The activities of the vestibular nerve were evaluated by counting the spikes of spontaneous discharge. The activities of the vestibular nerve were classified into regular, irregular, and intermediate types. Among 15 nerves that responded to stimulation of the horizontal semicircular canal, these three types of activity were observed in five each. The activity was elevated in four of the five nerves of the regular type by the application of positive pressure and decreased by reduction of the pressure (Fig. 10.19a). The same response pattern was observed in

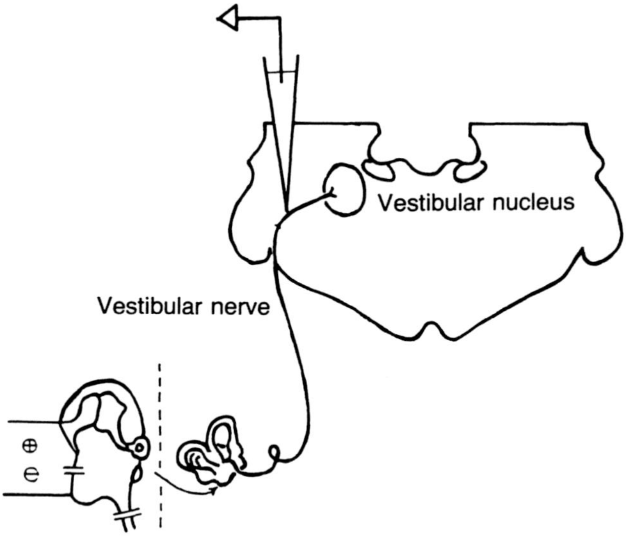

Fig. 10.18. Schema of experiment

two of the five nerves with the intermediate type, and one of the five showed increased activity when the pressure was both increased and decreased. Five nerves of the irregular type, one of the regular type, and two of the intermediate type did not respond to any changes in the middle ear pressure (Fig. 10.19b).

Among 14 vestibular nerves that responded to stimulation of the anterior semicircular canal, one (intermediate type) showed decreased activity with positive pressure, and one showed increased activity with negative pressure, but the remaining 13 did not respond to changes in the middle ear pressure (Fig. 10.20a). None of the 11 nerves that responded to stimulation of the posterior semicircular canal responded to the changes in middle ear pressure (Fig. 10.20b). The above results are summarized in Table 10.1.

These results support the assumption that changes in middle ear pressure influence the inner ear via the round and oval windows. Densert et al. (1986) recently observed changes in the perilymphatic pressure in cats while changing the middle ear pressure. Whether these changes in the perilymphatic pressure affect the activity of the hair cells of the inner ear is not known. However, the association between the changes in the vestibular nerve activity and those in the middle ear pressure suggests a route from the middle ear through the perilymphatic space and hair cells to the vestibular nerve.

Table 10.1. Responses of vestibular nerves to middle ear pressure loading

	Positive pressure			Negative pressure		
	Horizontal	Anterior	Posterior	Horizontal	Anterior	Posterior
Increased	7/15	0/15	0/11	1/15	1/15	0/11
Decreased	0/15	1/15	0/11	6/15	0/15	0/11
Unchanged	8/15	14/15	11/11	8/15	14/15	11/11

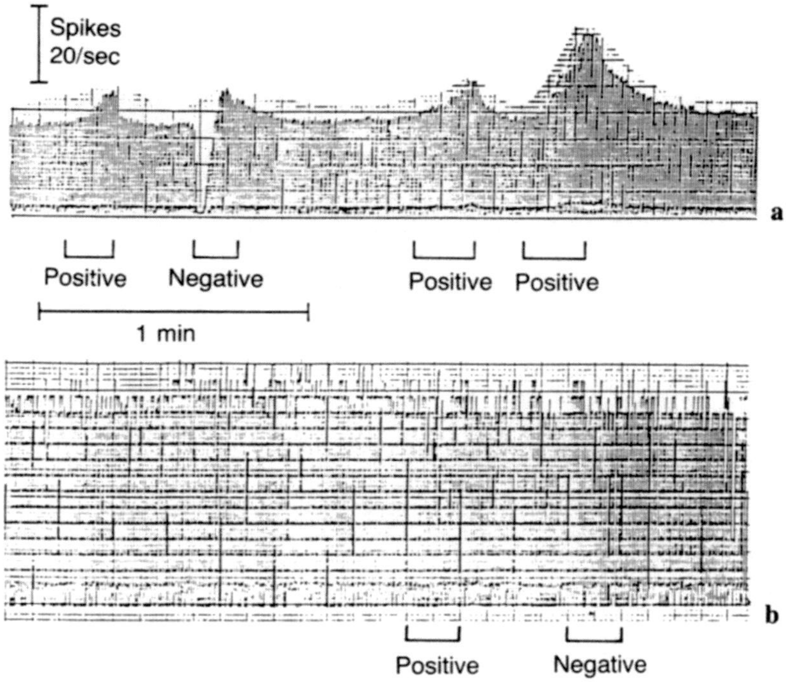

Fig. 10.19a, b. Effects of middle ear pressure on vestibular nerve activities (stimulation of horizontal semicircular canal). **a** Regular type; **b** intermediate type nerve

In this experiment, the vestibular nerves that responded to stimulation of the horizontal semicircular canal showed marked responses to the pressure changes, but those that responded to the vertical canal showed little response. Ingelstedt et al. (1974) altered the middle ear pressure of 79 healthy individuals in a pressure chamber, and observed transient nystagmus in five. These five subjects showed only horizontal nystagmus. This finding is in good agreement with the present results that pressure changes in the middle ear affected the horizontal semicircular canal but had little effect on the vertical canal. As changes in the middle ear pressure affect sway of the head and the center of gravity, responses to stimuli via the otolithic system should also be evaluated in future.

10.4.2 Summary

The effect of middle ear pressure on equilibrium was studied in 50 subjects consisting of OME patients and normal individuals, and its effect on vestibular nerve activity was studied in 13 cats. The results were as follows.

a) Negative middle ear pressure observed in patients with OME was found to affect equilibrium.
b) Middle ear pressure affected vestibular nerve activity. Generally, the activity increased or decreased with increasing or decreasing pressure, respectively.

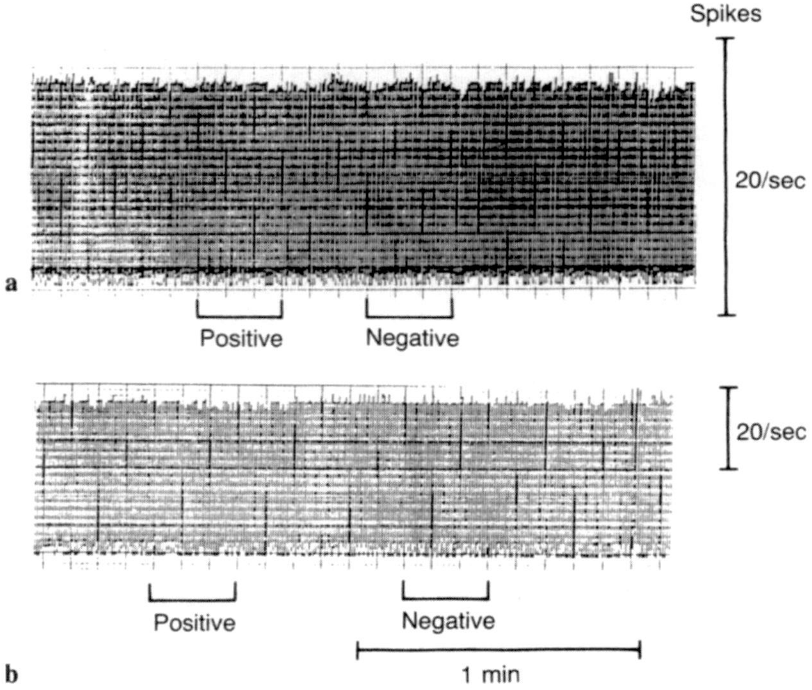

Fig. 10.20a, b. Effects of middle ear pressure on vestibular nerve activities. Stimulation of **a** anterior semicircular canal and **b** posterior semicircular canal

c) The horizontal semicircular canal is the most sensitive to middle ear pressure.
d) The probable route for middle ear pressure to affect the vestibulum was considered to be from the middle ear via the perilymph and hair cells of the inner ear to the vestibular nerve.

10.5 Summary of Chapter

Negative middle ear pressure as observed in OME patients exerted adverse effects not only on the middle ear but also on inner ear function. Although responses of the inner ear to the pressure change in the middle ear are not always consistent, the present study provided some clues to this rather complicated problem between the middle and inner ear.

It is almost certain, however, that negative middle ear pressure causes a reduction in bone conduction in the low-tone range due to temporary dysfunction of the cochlea. It is suggested that middle ear pressure influences the inner ear via one or both of the window that open into the inner ear.

A negative middle ear pressure was also found to affect equilibrium, and changes in equilibrium were shown to be mediated by the vestibular system. Studies in this area involve a number of difficulties, including instability of responses. However, further advances in the investigations are anticipated by clarification of the relation between middle ear pressure and the otolithic system or vestibular nerve nuclei as well as by the measurement of endolymphatic and perilymphatic pressure

References

Densert B, Densert O, Erlandsson B, Sheppard H (1986) Transmission of square wave pressure pulses through the perilymphatic fluid in cats. Acta Otolaryngol 102: 186–193

Fowler EP (1920) Drum tension and middle ear air pressures: Their determination, significance and effect upon the hearing. Ann Otol Rhinol Laryngol 29: 688–694

Fukuda T (1984) Statokinetic reflexes in equilibrium and movement. University of Tokyo Press, Tokyo

Ingelstedt S, Ivarsson A, Tjernström O (1974) Vertigo due to relative overpressure in the middle ear: An experimental study in man. Acta Otolaryngol 78: 1–14

Rahm EW Jr, Strother WF, Lucchina G, Gulick WL (1958) The effects of air pressure on the ear. Ann Otol Rhinol Laryngol 67: 170–177

Sawashima M (1957) Experimental study on bone conduction with impaired mobility at the oval and the round window. J Otolaryngol Jpn 61: 86–95 (in Japanese with English abstract)

Snider Rs, Niemer Wt (1961) A stereotaxic atlas of the cat brain. University of Chicago Press, Chicago

Tonndorf J, Tabor JR (1962) Closure of the cochlear windows: Its effect upon air- and bone-conduction. Ann Otol Rhinol Laryngol 71: 5–29

Wever Eg, Bray CW, Lawrence M (1972) The effects of pressure in the middle ear. J Exp Psychol 30: 40–52

Subject Index

Made in the USA
Las Vegas, NV
02 December 2024

13240943R00112